EMS2
THE LIFE OF YOUR JOB

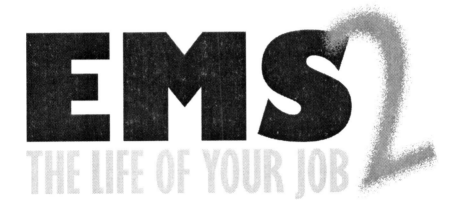

DEVIN KERINS

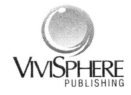

VIVISPHERE
PUBLISHING

ISBN-10: 1-58776-149-1
ISBN-13: 978-1-58776-149-2

Printed in the United States of America

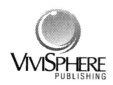

VIVISPHERE PUBLISHING
A division of NetPub Corporation
675 Dutchess Turnpike, Poughkeepsie, NY 12603
www.vivisphere.com   (800) 724-1100

THANK YOU

This book couldn't have been possible without the support and help of a lot of people. Forgive me if I forgot anyone or misspelled your names:

Wendell Green, Jay Field, JJ Johnson, Rich Neurouter, John Cruz, Joe Crouchman, Henry Solares, Barry Fitzpatrick, Meg Chandler, Tito and Shauna Rodriguez, Nancy and Julio Rivera, Liza Rivera, Mike Carrig, Chris Fink, Mike Alessi, Matt Testino, Jay Bowles, Tim Phelan, Rich Gorman, Norman Brown, Ralph Bravo, Oscar Santella, Vanessa and Fred Siverio, Carmella Tatum, Darnell Gourdine, Nilda Baez, Pedro Leon, Bill Newby, Greg Bulger, Corrine Hernandez, Myra Stith, Martin Kalski, Dave Aromin, Vince Froncek, Tarrance Byrant, Derek Lyon, Virginia Ferrera, Mickie and Joe Slattery, Harvey Weber, Jose Aviles, Vinnie Glenn, Ricardo Reyes, Chris Marcinak, Nick Randisi, Bill Castagno, Bob Casey, Bill Reiner, Eric Fortmann, Pablo Lopez, Bo Pitts John Syzmanek, Sandi Sanderson, Victor and Elaina Cook, Jimmy and Sosa, Elvia Lopez, Vinnie Cheng, Joe Vallo, Mike Yeh, Don Heath, Marc Poveromp Anne and Scott Stein, Meggin Stein, Carol Bastian, O'Dea Parson, Chris Dimeglio, Randy Wagner, Dave Burns, Mike Burns, Kevin Reading Sr and Jr, Ray Nagy, Andrew Condrat, the guys at Station 23 in Lawrenceville, Scott Bahner, Dan Dolphin, the guys at Medic

17/Engine 36/Ladder 20 in Philadelphia, the gang at Squad 129 in Lawrenceville,

George Fiero of GNF Enterprises in Union City, NJ and Joe Guido of The Village Barbershop in Lawrenceville, NJ for being my unofficial public relations guys, and Vivisphere editor, Kevin Ahearn.

Those closest to me: Bill and Cris Maloney, Erin Belz, my family: Dad, Sean, Brendan, Brian, Trish, Patrick, and Mom (still with me), and the love of my life Antoinette Jensen and Cassandra.

CONTENTS

9/11/2002

I'm standing on the pier at Exchange Place looking out across the Hudson River at a New York City skyline that now seems naked. Exactly one year since the Towers fell, and I still have yet to get used to the skyline without them.

The 9-11 Memorial Committee has organized an emotional ceremony to commemorate the day that forever changed our lives. My partner and I stand in the crowd with people from all walks of life and listen to the speeches, poems, and songs that those gathered have written.

The Committee has arranged for one white dove to be released into the air for each resident of Jersey City who died in the attack. I well up with tears as they read off the names and a police officer plays *Taps* on a bugle. Then, the moment they have been building up to, the Committee releases the birds into the air.

Something has gone wrong. Only half of the birds are able to fly. The rest plunge into the Hudson River. Of those that could fly, most carelessly defecate on the Parking Authority personnel who have gathered, arousing a loud cheer from the attendees. I watch in disbelief as a rouge bird flies directly at my partner and me. At the last moment, the dove banks to the left and flies into the side of the office building we are standing next to. I watch as he slides down the glass and remains motionless.

"Dude," my partner says, "I think he's dead."

Right on cue, the bird scrambles to his feet. I raise my hands in triumph and exclaim, "He's okay!" The people around me cheer again.

As I spend the next half-hour fishing doves out the Hudson River, one thought keeps creeping into my mind – *It must be me!* Even at such a somber occasion, I still attract the strange and unusual.

September 11th, 2001 will forever be, in my mind, the day the world found out why emergency service personnel do their jobs. The world saw images of heroic firefighters and police officers rushing into the World Trade Center to save lives. The world saw images of EMTs and paramedics rendering care to an overwhelming number of patients. And for the first time that I can recall, we were looked upon as heroes, as people to look up to.

Little children began to see "ordinary," hardworking individuals as something to aspire to be, instead of just looking up to sports figures. At an event stand a few months later, a group of kids asked me for my autograph.

People saw the reason for our job. We rush in when everyone else rushes out. We, a select few number of people, have dedicated ourselves to risking our lives so that others may live. It's not an easy job, and it's certainly not for everyone.

The turnover rate for EMTs and paramedics is high. Many only stay for a few short years – using the job as a springboard to get ahead in other fields. Some go on to become doctors or nurses or other higher paying positions within the medical field. Others use the teamwork and leadership skills they learned on the job to go on to completely unrelated fields. It seems that only a small number make a career out of it. I've been doing this for almost ten years. At age 26, I am often looked upon as a "dinosaur." I feel like one when I tell newer guys who are older than I am how we did things when I started. "Back in my day..."

There are any number of reasons why EMTs burn out quickly: the ever present-fear of being sued, the stress of dealing with management, health care reforms, and a variety of other restrictions that constantly hinder us from doing the job the way we wish we could. Add to that the stress of knowing that you'll most likely come home late from every shift, if you come home at all.

Why would anyone want to stay in such a stressful and dangerous job? The answer to that becomes clear to me a few hours after the morning's 9-11 ceremonies.

The Committee has also planned to have a free concert in Liberty State Park. We've been called in to stand by at the event, which is expected to attract thousands, as well as celebrities and politicians of all sorts. In accordance with the way the day seems to be going, nothing is going right for the concert people. To top things off, the wind has picked up and is threatening to blow the stage over. They cancel the concert, but the EMTs are stuck in the park until the stage is taken apart.

With nothing to do and left up to our own devices, we have to amuse ourselves. Conversation starts up with gossip and making fun of each other. Occasionally someone throws in a "war" story, which is then countered by another person trying to outdo the other. I look up from the mindless banter in time to see someone slip a sandwich unnoticed into the lapel of the current speaker's jacket. We try not to laugh and see how long he'll go without noticing the sandwich on his shoulder.

This carries on into the evening. We watch the sun set behind the Statue of Liberty together. Then, beneath the stars, our conversation turns to a tearful remembrance of friends lost in the attacks. The tears don't last as long as they used to, and for the first time in a year, we agree that we've begun to feel "normal" again.

Though things will never be the same, we have learned to lean on each other in hard times. EMS has always been a tight community, but following the attacks, we've become even closer. It's that camaraderie that allows us to go to work everyday with a smile on our faces. It's what allows us to tease each other relentlessly without hurting feelings. It's what forms bonds between partners that make us almost as strong as brothers. It's what creates memories like these that will stay with us for a lifetime and keeps us coming back for more.

HOW WE GOT HERE

"One day I'm going to write a book about this!"

I can't tell you how many times I've heard that. During my first six years in Emergency Medical Services, I must have said it myself three times a day. I think back to swapping stories with coworkers till three in the morning over a greasy diner table. I couldn't help but get good at it, putting just the spin on a tale to grab their attention. I began to believe that if my coworkers liked the way I told stories, then maybe other people would too.

I *was* going to write a book about EMS. But I kept putting it off for one reason after another. Then one November when I was 20, the doctor gave me the news. My hard of hearing I had attributed to loud rock music and four years of ambulance sirens had been caused by a tumor. If left untreated, it could spread to my brain. I endured two painful surgeries and recoveries, and so far everything has been good. The ordeal had a silver lining: it left me with a sense of my own mortality. It was a fluke that I even took the hearing test that had revealed the tumor. If I had put that off, things would have been a lot worse.

Stuck at home to recover, I had the perfect excuse to start the book. Enough opportunities in my life had already passed me by. Besides, I had nothing else to do. I couldn't watch the same movie over and over again. My parents had just bought a new dog, so all the sympathy I would have gotten was channeled into doting over Nugget.

I had no real idea how to write a book, but I wanted to keep it light, and I had to make it real. EMS, like police and firefighters, is an "us" and "them" organization. My book had to have "us" written all the way through it. Full of bravery and heroism? The problem with telling an heroic story is that people tend to think you're making yourself out to be someone you're not – even if it really happened the way you said it did. I'd stick with the truth, but concentrate on the funny and unusual and there was plenty of both.

I returned to work after surgery with a mission. Coworkers found out I was writing a book and stories flowed more freely.

"I can't offer you any money," I'd tell my sources. "

That's okay," all replied. "I've got a great one nobody will believe!"

I needed a title. *You Can't Make This Shit Up!* was my first choice, but that would never play in the mall. *View From the Street* was my second stab. To maintain its realistic tone, I would only write while at work, spending many a shift in the front of my ambulance or in a quiet corner of the station with my laptop, thinking about old calls and taking long trips down Memory Lane.

Before I knew it, my masterpiece was done. Or so I thought. I wrote letters to some 30 literary agents to get them interested in selling the book. Almost all of them wrote back rejecting me.

"There's no market for it." One said.

Another said, "There are already too many books like it out there."

A couple of other agents offered to read my book if I paid them a fee. That was never an option. If the book couldn't speak for itself, then it probably didn't deserve to be published.

Just when I was about to give up, I got an email from an agent who was confident we could sell my book with a few "revisions." I spent the next year or so with my new agent/editor getting the right feel for the book. He had never been involved with EMS before. If I could keep him reading, then I could hold the interest of people not in EMS. That would expand my reading audience, sell more books, and put me in the lap of luxury. So the last part never happened? But like Meatloaf sang, "Two outa three ain't bad."

All polished up, *EMS: The Job of Your Life* was submitted to a dozen publishers. And rejected by every one.

My agent was used to it. He was new to the business and still looking for his first sale. Oh great, I thought, I've never written a book and he's never sold one. What a team! But then I realized that would make for a great success story if or when I made it big.

Such are the dreams of wannabe writers. Just when I thought it would never be, my agent e-mailed me, "Send your manuscript overnight to this company!"

Off it went on Thursday, and on Monday…Yes!

VIVISPHERE Publishing was a small company, but size didn't matter in this case—*EMS: The Job of Your Life* was going to be a book!

I couldn't wait to tell my mom. She had just gone into the hospital for a routine surgery. As soon as she was awake, I showed her my publishing contract. Still weak from her surgery, my biggest supporter gave me the biggest Mom-hug I'd ever received.

"Maybe now you'll let me read it!" she said.

I had kept the manuscript from her because of the profanity and the sex injury chapter. "Heaven forgive you!" I imagined her saying again and again. But now that my pile of paper was going to be a real book...I rushed home to print a copy for her to read. She never did. Her condition worsened during the night and she never came off the ventilator. As I sit here writing the sequel, I get the feeling she's reading *EMS II: The Life of Your Job* over my shoulder and can almost hear her screaming, "Heaven forgive you!" That must mean I'm onto something good.

Because nothing can be easy for me, small-time publishing came with big problems. I had hoped for some help marketing the book, but for the longest time I had to do the "new author thing" and sell the book myself. When my first sales figures came in, I could put a name to every book sold. "Oh yeah, Mike bought one. Jay bought two..."

Slowly, almost torturously, the book caught on. My crowning moment came at work when someone I had never met before stopped me and said, "I loved your book. I got three of my friends to buy it. I got it in the truck. Would you autograph it?"

In no time at all, I was carrying the 'Official Book Signing Sharpie' to work and autographing a book after almost every call. It was an amazing feeling—I had become an EMT somebody!

"Bro, I loved your book! When's the next one coming out?" Hearing that felt almost as good as saving a life. I was going to write a *second* book!

So here we are again. Ready for another foray into the world of madness and emergency medicine? If this is your second ride with me, welcome back. If this is your first time out, just suspend all disbelief and abandon your preconceived notions of reality and common sense - they'll only get in the way.

(To save time and fill the book with more fun and frivolity, I've omitted a glossary. If you've never been on an ambulance and find yourself lost, please refer to the glossary in my first book. If you don't have it, jump on Amazon and buy a copy. Hey, I gotta make more money somehow!)

Once again, I remind you that the views and thoughts expressed in this book are not those of the organizations to which I am affiliated. To my knowledge, all the stories are true, but I did change some locations and names to protect the innocent, the guilty, and those lacking in common sense.

Enough of this intro, the dispatcher's calling us. Let's go snatch back some lives from the greedy clutches of death.

A DAY IN THE
LIFE AND DEATH

I sit on a towel looking over the Caribbean Sea, feeling the sand between my toes and smelling the salty sea air. The air is mixed with the scent of her shampoo. I hold her in my arms as we look out across the island, watching the sun come up over the palm trees and resort hotels.

It's daybreak on the equator and life is good. I bring her close as the sun pushes its way through what few clouds there are and bathes the land with a red glow. A few birds fly low overhead. I run my hands through her curly brown hair.

She gets up, takes me by the hand, and leads me to the crystal blue waters. We embrace and fall in to the water. We kiss and...

Thump, thump, thump

"Excuse me! Hey buddy, *excuse me*! Do you have some spare change to help a brother out?" The thumping on the window and the sight of the disheveled man outside my ambulance snap me back into reality with such a jolt that I slam my knees against the dashboard.

Ouch, that'll leave a mark!

"I said," he continues despite my attempts to ignore him, "you got any spare change?"

"No. Now please go away."

"C'mon man. You know who I am. You know me. Tell ya what, I'll help you out if you help me out."

I look around and get my bearings. *I have to stop working double shifts. Twenty-four hours of this!* I'm sitting in the passenger seat of my ambulance in a rundown part of town. My partner is nowhere to be found. He must have run into his house to get something. I wish he would have warned me instead of letting me sleep. Something always happens when I try to catch a nap. Now Donald is outside of my window asking for money.

Sure I know Donald. I've been picking him up for a few years. He's a junkie; heroin's his favorite. I look at the street corner and marvel that it's a little far south in the city for him to be hanging out. Geography doesn't matter much now; he's standing in front of my window begging.

Not thinking too clearly because I'm still groggy from my nap, I roll down the window. He sticks his hand inside and gestures to shake my hand. Thinking it's a mistake, yet somehow powerless to stop myself, I shake his hand. It feels cold and grimy. *I'll be obsessing about that all day.*

Suddenly, he pulls his hand back and starts looking around suspiciously. "I know they're watching!"

"Who?" *Why am I even engaging in this conversation? Just give him the money and get him out of here!*

"See, I'm putting my life in danger by talking to the am'lance. They're watching. Do you see them?" I've learned by now not to answer that question and just act like I don't hear him. "See, I just gotsta keep looking at them to see the signals they're putting out. You know the signals, right?"

I try to ignore him, but it becomes obvious very quickly that I can't. He starts making all of these outrageous gestures and telling me what each one means. "And if they want to 'waste' you, they make a big 'W' like this..."

I stare at the radio in hopes that the dispatcher will pick up on my telepathic signals and give me a call. An eternity seems to pass and no call comes. *Why should it? One never comes when you really want one, only when you don't.*

"Look, Donald, if I give you some change will you leave me alone?"

He stops abruptly and looks at me with delight. "Sure."

"Then here." I dig into my pocket and pull out a handful of change from my soda fund. Without counting it, I hand it to him.

"I'll pay you back. I just want to get some chips or something to eat."

"Whatever." *I know he's just going to hit up someone else until he has enough money to shoot up and I'll probably have to come back to pick him up later.*

As he walks away, I roll up the window and find something good to listen to on the radio. *All I wanted was a quick power nap to get ready for my night shift.* I get comfortable and settle in for another nap. I've been working all day and I now I have to work tonight to earn a little overtime. A few minutes of sleep should get me charged up enough to make through the night. I close my eyes and...

"Unit Three-Zero-Nine, I have a job for you."

Great, why couldn't they have called a couple of minutes ago?

"Go ahead," I grumble into the mike.

"Ocean and Orient, that's Ocean Avenue and Orient Avenue, on the outside, for the violent female armed with a knife. Do not go off without police."

Heck of a way to start off the second half of this tour, but I'll take it nonetheless. Emotionally disturbed persons, especially females with weapons, are always fun.

"Three–Zero–Nine received, Ocean and Orient. On the way."

I look out and see my partner jogging across the street with a smile on his face. "Sorry I took so long." He hands me some tin foil trays that smell absolutely wonderful. "Midnight snack." *His wife must have been cooking again.* My stomach starts to do back flips, begging me to feed it what's in the tray.

Unfortunately, I'll have to wait until later.

My partner puts the truck in drive and pulls out into traffic. "Hey, did you see Donald down here?"

"Yeah, I saw him," I groan as I frantically wipe my hands with a sterile napkin. I let out a sigh as I watch the scenery I've seen so many times before pass by. *Another day, another dollar, and more adventures to be experienced.*

OCEAN AND ORIENT

19:05 hours

As we approach the intersection where we're supposed to find our patient, I see a petite lady leaning against a chain link fence. It looks as though she has something in her left hand, and she is frantically rubbing it against her right wrist. There's no police on scene yet, but I feel in the mood to take my chances for some reason. I give a wail on the siren. Surprised, she throws the object over the fence and walks towards us.

She lifts her hands so her palms are towards me. "Do you see what they did to me?" She has scratches on her right wrist.

"Who?"

She motions to a group of people standing by a house on the corner. "Them!"

I look towards them; they look back at me with equal bewilderment. "What did they do that with ma'am?" I'm trying my best to be patient.

"A bottle or something."

"You mean this?" My partner calls from the other side of the fence. He has a crushed soda can in his hands. He had seen where she threw it when we pulled up. That almost makes up for letting me wake up to Donald rapping on my window. *Almost!*

"Yeah, that's it!"

Not wanting to argue, and being very intrigued as to where this is going, I press on. "Why did they do that?"

"Cuz they're sticking up for him!"

"Him who?"

"My, ah, ex-boyfriend. He tried to rape me!"

So this is getting a little serious now. Whether or not she's telling the truth, I have to get the police involved. *And boy, am I glad I do!*

After a few minutes of frustratingly trying to interview our patient while we wait for the cops, the first radio car arrives.

"What's the problem?" The police officer asks. When he looks at my patient, an expression of recognition crosses his face. "Oh, never mind. I think I know already. I'll be back in a few." He slams the ambulance door and walks towards the crowd.

A few moments later he returns. He opens the door and yells in. "Sharon (*I'm surprised he knows her name since she never told us*), for the last time, it's not rape if he pays you eight bucks for it!"

Her head snaps back in shock, I drop my pen, and my partner fumbles to get the words out. "Wh–what do you mean?"

"You guys don't know Sharon? She's one of our regulars. Always pulling this crap. She gives this guy a little some-thing-something, he gives her eight bucks for it, and she says that she was raped. Am I right?"

She looks down at the floor and says nothing at first. Then she shows the officer her wrists. "Well, look what he did to me tonight!"

"You guys have a good night," I say to the officer as I step out and close the door.

As I drive to the hospital, I laugh to myself that even this amazes me.

COMMUNITY EDUCATION AND OUTREACH

One of my favorite aspects of EMS is educating the public. It gives me the chance to interact with people in a more relaxed environment, (Hopefully no one in the class is having a heart attack!) and to share my knowledge in hopes that others will benefit from it. If I can help one person in the group, then it'll be worth it.

Community education doesn't always occur within a classroom setting. It can happen on calls. I try to make public service announcements whenever possible. Educating today's youth so that they will not become future patients is my mission. However, that plan often goes awry and they wind up becoming stories.

Dispatched on a summer afternoon, when I arrived, the fire department first responders were already on scene, along with a large group of kids. The patient who was supposed to be "unconscious and unresponsive" was sitting up on the steps of a house.

"What's the problem ma'am?" As soon as I asked the question I caught a whiff of her and had a strong suspicion what her answer would be.

"What do you think is wrong?" She answered back with a sarcastic tone. "I'm drunk!"

I tried to help her up but a young boy from the crowd ran up to me. "Mista, mista. She's got rocks in her mouth!"

"Rocks?" I asked and he nodded. Thinking that he meant crack cocaine, I told her to open her mouth — a nauseating mistake. When she did I saw four of the most disgusting teeth that I had ever seen in my life - and only four. Fighting back a dry heave, I said to the kid, "Those aren't rocks."

"Yes they are." He said insistently. "I seen 'em myself!"

"Those aren't rocks, trust me."

"Yes they are. I know they are."

"Look, kid. Do you remember what the rocks looked like?"

"Yeah, they were small and pointy and black."

"Good. Then you will always remember to brush your teeth."

The look on his face at the moment of comprehension was priceless. He screamed his disgust and ran off down the street. My first public service announcement.

The police were on the scene when I arrived for a young girl who had fallen and cut her hand. The officers told me that the patient, who was 14, and her friend, who was 15, had been drinking when the patient fell.

The girls were giggling and having a great time. The police officer told them that he never wanted to see them drinking again. They laughed at him, and I would too. The chances of him running into them again, or remembering them when he did, were very slim. What kind of a threat is that?

The whole way to the hospital, the girls were giggling and laughing about the officer. Now I felt it was civic duty to set these girls on the right path.

When we arrived at the hospital, I took them into the ER waiting area. I quickly looked around and found what I needed. An hour earlier we had brought in one of our regular drunks. He was particularly nasty today, in both attitude and stench.

I sat the girls down next to him and bet them they would move in 60 seconds. They laughed at me, but sat next to him. In less than 60 seconds, they were across the room and gagging from the stench. I told them to take a good look at the drunk and remember him, because that's how they might wind up in a few years. *Dramatic? Perhaps. But maybe they'll consider drinking responsibly later in life.*

The fire company that I belong to runs a popular fire prevention and safety program for grammar school kids. The star of the program is Flashy the Fire Dog, a giant stuffed Dalmatian that sits in a remote controlled fire truck. One instructor stands in another room and controls Flashy. He has a headset and when he talks, Flashy's mouth and head move like *he* is talking. Another instructor stands with Flashy, talking to the kids and relaying their questions to the microphone in Flashy's ear. The kids love it.

One day they decided to let me control Flashy at a community picnic. I was doing well, keeping up as best I could with the kids. Then, something went wrong.

Suddenly, Flashy's head jammed. I could only turn the head to the right. I couldn't look at the kids on my left. The instructor became a little annoyed that Flashy wasn't looking at the kids. "Hey Flashy, let's not be rude," he said. "Look at the kids when you are talking to them."

I didn't know what to do. Flashy wouldn't budge. "Ah, my neck really hurts. I was up late last night fighting a fire."

"Flashy, don't be silly. Just look at the kids."

"I can't. I really can't!"

The instructor still had no idea what was going on. "Flashy, look at the kids or I'll put you back in the doghouse!"

I gave up and did the only thing that I could. I spun the head around backwards like something out of *The Exorcist.* The kids ran off screaming and crying. For some reason – I can't put my finger on it – they wouldn't let me control Flashy any more.

I'm not the only one who had a problem with Flashy. Another firefighter was operating him when he noticed that the batteries in the remote were running low. Trying to head off disaster, he turned the head of the dog towards his partner and said, "Mike, Mike, I don't feel so good. I think I need to go home."

"Nonsense, Flashy," said the instructor and continued to carry on with his lecture.

Noticing the controls weren't responding, he pleaded again, "Mike, I think I'm going to have a seizure."

With that, the dog took on a life of its own and started spinning out of control. It knocked over two children before running over a teacher and ramming into a wall.

Another annual public relations show we like to do every year is "Operation Santa." One of the firefighters dresses up like Santa and we go around the district spreading holiday cheer and giving out candy canes. It's always fun and we have a great time. One year I went to step off the fire truck to deliver some candy, slipped on the ice, and fell flat on my ass. Another year, a group of us were talking trash to each other and a candy cane fight erupted.

Part of delivering this holiday cheer involves visiting the nursing homes with Santa. The residents love it, and it's a good feeling to see how appreciative they are. One lady was way too appreciative.

Bill, a firefighter, had given her a candy cane, and wished

her a merry Christmas. She immediately began telling everyone that Bill was her boyfriend. She followed us all around the nursing home, holding his arm, and kissing him on the cheek. She even went as far as to invite him to stay the night.

"I can't do that," Bill tried as gently as possible to decline. "My mother won't let me."

"Hey, Bill," I said, loud enough to get her attention as I picked up a phone then hung it up. "That was your mom on the phone. She said it's all right."

The lady got this big smile on her face and hugged him tighter. "Ma'am," another firefighter said, "show me what room you're in so we can move another bed in there." Bill's face was getting very red.

"That won't be necessary," she looked at Bill lovingly, "he can share mine!"

We all cracked up and took pictures of the happy couple as Bill swore he would kill us.

Don't think for a moment the abuse stopped there. Oh, no! We enlarged some of the photos to poster size and hung them up around the firehouse, the first aid squad where he was a member, and at the local hospitals. It feels great when I'm not on the receiving end of everyone's jokes.

I agreed to volunteer at a senior citizen's health fair. I was having a great time, taking blood pressures, talking, and enjoying free food. There were other booths, offering free body fat analysis, foot analysis, and hearing tests.

My friend Alexis persuaded me to take advantage. The first booth I went to was the body fat analysis. I couldn't believe my score. It was a lot better than I expected. *No, I will not tell what it is! Gotta have some secrets, don't I?*

Next the eyesight exam. I know I can't see, but the test showed that my eyesight had gotten a lot worse. Great, I have a good body fat ratio, but can't see.

After that the hearing test. I had always suspected that I was beginning to have trouble hearing, even at age twenty. I sat down and the lady placed the headphones on my head. "I'll start with the right ear. Just let me know when you hear a sound." She began playing with some buttons and looking up at me. After about two minutes of total silence, she said, "Okay, now we'll move onto the left ear. And, by the way, here's my business card."

At this point, I had a decent body fat ratio, but I was deaf in one ear and blind. I was down, but it was time to get kicked even more. Time for the foot screening.

I figured, "What the hell, might as well." After all, I was sure I had no problems with my feet.

I sat down and the podiatrist began examining my foot. After a few moments he got up and said, "Okay, I know what the problem is."

Know what the problem is? That would imply that there is a problem to know about. I have no problem with my feet! Apparently I do. It won't bother me until I am older, but there is something wrong with my feet.

Can't see, can't hear, and I have deformed feet. *This was one of those days I wished I had stayed in bed!*

Serving the public in a non-medical way sometimes becomes part of the job. I have no problem helping an elderly person back into bed every now and then, or fixing a problem in the house that would prevent future injuries. But sometimes, this service gets taken advantage of.

All it takes is for one EMT to be overly helpful and that's the end of it. My friend was dispatched for a fall victim. When he arrived he found an elderly lady lying on the floor. She had been trying to get to bathroom when she fell. She asked if that could help her back into her wheelchair. The crew did so. Then she asked if they could help her into the bathroom. Going against their better judgment, they did so. They helped her go to the bathroom and helped back into bed. Supposedly, there was a home health aide who would be around in the morning to help her. She signed a refusal that she didn't want to go to the hospital and they were on their way.

Three hours later, she called back because she needed to go to the bathroom again. This time, they helped her, but were not so nice about it. She signed a refusal, and they were on their way.

Three hours later, she called again. This time, my friend's supervisor also responded and made her go to the hospital.

That is not an isolated incident. An ambulance was dispatched for a similar call in Jersey City. They assisted the man into the bathroom, got him to sign a refusal and left. Now this man calls all the time. If he needs a glass of water, he calls an ambulance. If he needs his fan fixed, he calls 911. Cats need to be fed? *911.* Can't reach the thermostat? *911.* Can't reach his medicine? *Where's the ambulance?* He must know that it is New Jersey law that no one can be denied an ambulance if they request one, so he doesn't bother lying anymore. He says exactly what he wants.

If you, the reader, want to do something to endear yourself to the hearts of EMS personnel around the country and insure prompt medical attention, rally Congress for a law that would allow us to *refuse* to send an ambulance to people like this.

Am I insensitive when I say I won't help some people? What I mean is that I'll help someone back into bed. I'll even go as far to carry someone up a flight of stairs if I know that this won't become a regular occurrence. My pet peeve is someone calling for an ambulance because they need help going to the bathroom. This will always result in me forcing the person to go to the hospital. If a person can't go to the bathroom on his or her own, someone needs to start considering a home health aid. *Nothing forces the issue more than an expensive hospital bill and an extended emergency room visit just so that someone can wipe your butt!*

My partner and I responded for a fall victim. When we arrived, a little old lady met us at the door. She apologized for calling us and said that she only did it because she couldn't get her husband back into bed. I said it was no problem. *Hell, I'd rather spend all day lifting people back into bed than carrying them down the stairs.*

We found the husband on the floor next to the bed. He was big, but it was a cake job. We put him back on the bed and had him sign a refusal. The wife then asked us if there was any way we could fix the bed. It was slumping down to one side and it causes her bedridden husband to fall off.

"Not a problem!" My partner said as he climbed under the bed. He's the Mr. Fix-it of the two of us, so I let him do his thing. He came up a few minutes later and the bed was fixed. The wife thanked us and offered us some iced tea, which we gratefully accepted. While the other ambulances were running around answering calls, we hung around for a few minutes talking with the lady.

We decided it was time to leave, said our good byes and thank you's and left. "They seemed like a nice couple," I said in passing to my partner as we got into the ambulance.

"Don't be fooled. There's freaky shit going on that house."

"What do you mean?"

"The only way the bed gets like that is if there is some serious monkey lovin' happening on it."

I am certain that that image will cause some sort of problem with my love life.

One night, after responding to half a dozen "baby with a fever" calls in a row I was pissed off. The patient's mother met us at the door, then proceeded to walk back up three long flights of stairs. After walking up – thinking to myself all the while how it can't be a good sign that I'm twenty four and feeling my pulse in my eyeballs – I followed her into a bedroom where she sat down on the bed and started playing with the baby.

"What's the problem?"

"We were at the hospital earlier today and they sent him home with a fever of 101.5."

"So what's the problem?"

"It's now 102."

"Okay, and what's the problem?"

Now she was becoming extremely upset. "Well, it went up!"

I don't know why, but I wanted to see where I could take this. "It's not higher. Not really. It might be you're reading your thermometer wrong."

"102 is much higher than 101.5!"

"Did they give you medicine to take?"

"They told me to get Children's Tylenol."

"Did you?"

"No."

Then I asked the question that is guaranteed to make anyone upset in this situation. "What do you want the hospital to do for you?"

"Oh, what? I'm supposed to let my baby sit here and die?"

Obviously I was upsetting her, but boy was she getting me good. The baby had been running this fever all day. She called for the ambulance and had to wait some time because we were busy taking other babies with fevers to the hospital. Yet she waited until *now* to start getting everything together. It took her ten minutes to get the child's things together. In that time three life threatening emergencies were dispatched. Two of which we would have been closer to had we not been dealing with her.

"Ma'am, are you ready?"

"Just a minute."

"Okay, take your time. It's not like there are real emergencies right around the corner from here."

Have you ever wondered why it takes so long to get an ambulance sometimes? I hope this clears it up for you.

CITY GENERAL HOSPITAL
EMERGENCY ROOM

19:20 Hours

I park the truck in the only space that is available. I count six ambulances parked in the emergency room parking lot – the sign of a busy night ahead. I only did four calls during the first half of my double, so I know I'll be paying for it tonight.

I unlock the side door and try to coax my patient outside.

"No way!" She screams and folds her arms across her chest. "They gonna tie me down if I go in there!"

"Look, Sharon," I try to sound polite. "No one's going to tie you down unless you do something to deserve it." I extend my hand in a friendly gesture.

She studies my hand and for a second I think she'll actually follow me inside peacefully. *Wishful thinking!* She slaps my hand away and spits at me. "I'm not going in there!"

She's lucky she didn't hit me. I'm slowly turning into my alter ego – the "Not-so-nice" Devin. But I try to remain professional. "Sharon, why are you doing this to me? Wasn't I nice to you? Let's go."

She lets out an ear-piercing screech. "No! I ain't gonna be tied down!" She retreats as far against the bench seat as she can.

"Sharon, if you don't get the hell out of this truck *I'm* going to tie you down!" My partner grabs her by the arm and tries to get her to stand. She tries to swing at him with the other arm, but I stop it in time. I hold one arm, my partner takes the other, and we lead her out of the ambulance. Every few steps she purposely stumbles and we have to yank her to her feet.

There is a group of people huddled outside the ER doors, sharing a lighter for their cigarettes. It's an odd mix – two nurses, a doctor, a security guard, two paramedics, and a half a dozen civilians (presumably family members of patients inside). The paramedics give me a nod. The ER staff shakes their heads. The civilians give me an astonished look as I escort my patient inside. From their reaction, I can tell they have nothing to do with EMS

Predictably, City General Hospital's ER is packed. I wouldn't expect anything less on a Friday night in the summer. Inside, two EMS crews are cleaning off their stretchers with a spray bottle full of bleach. *Not a good sign.* Nurses and ER technicians move hurriedly through the room. It is a bustling ER. There is a loud buzz as dozens of conversations come together into one unintelligible cacophony. Above the noise, one sound is clear – a child wailing from the pediatric exam rooms. *No matter what hospital you go to, no matter what hour, there's always a kid wailing!*

We guide our patient to the front desk so the charge nurse can tell us where she wants us to place her. It's shift change, so finding a nurse to give a report to will be difficult. Four nurses sit in a semi-circle on the opposite side of the desk. In the center of them is a stack of charts and a list of patients on top of it. They mumble amongst themselves, seemingly oblivious to the sobbing patient my partner and I are supporting.

A shouting match breaks out and draws our attention the door to the waiting room. A young woman is yelling, demanding to see her boyfriend. An overweight, balding security guard tries to contain her. The nurses look up briefly from their conversation and I try to capitalize on it. "Excuse me," I say politely but to no avail.

"Dev," my partner says, "forget this, we know where's she going anyway." He's right. Patients who are intoxicated or having emotional crises go to the same area.

We begin to move down the corridor to the treatment room we plan to put her in. Along the way I catch a glimpse of the mess in the Trauma Room. A patient on a ventilator occupies one of the two beds. I can't tell if it's a male or a female because all I can see are feet. The other bed looks slightly out of place. It's neatly made, surrounded by a litter of bloody bandages and dirty, discarded equipment.

Next I pass the asthma room. Two patients, a young Hispanic girl and a gray haired black gentleman, look relaxed as they hold nebulizer treatments to their mouths, staring indifferently as the mist rises from the plastic tubes they are breathing from.

My patient begins screaming again. "I don't want to be tied down! You bastards can't do this to me!" She throws herself on the floor. We pick her up, her feet not touching the floor, and carry her the rest of the way. She kicks and curses in protest. A Middle Eastern family looks on in horror, the mother pulling her son close and uttering something in Arabic to him.

"Sorry, folks," I say with a smile, as we carry her by the family.

The room we want is at the end of the Emergency Room, tucked away from the other patients. Typical patients in this room include drunks, homeless people, violent patients, and those with odors that are less than tolerable – or patients who are a combination of all of the above. One such patient is in the bed against the far wall.

A disheveled man lies on his side; his pants still down around his ankles. Somehow his sheets have been pulled down, exposing his buttocks. One leg and one arm are in leather restraints – "two points" as we say in the biz. He doesn't appear to move as we enter the room. His odor does all the talking for him. It's a pungent blend – a mix of urine, sweat, and onion. There is something more to that odor, something so foul it can only be described as a decaying human flesh smell. Like burning flesh, it's a smell words cannot do justice, but an odor that you never forget.

A security guard heard the commotion our patient was making and comes in to help us. He is radioing for back up and telling someone to bring four point restraints. Sharon is being so uncooperative that all her extremities need to be restrained. Once reinforcements have arrived, each security guard grabs a limb and wrestles her onto the bed. She puts up on hell of a fight and as I wipe the sweat from my forehead I am thankful it's not me in there wrestling with her.

My partner tries to track down a nurse to sign our forms. In the meantime, I step outside and take a long, greedy sip from my ice cold water bottle.

The heat is becoming unbearable. Sweat is already dripping down the small of my back making me feel extremely uncomfortable. Soon, I know I'll forget it's there and go on about my business as usual. I turn the air conditioner on in the truck and feel the cool air freezing my perspiration.

I call back in service and get set for the next assignment.

CODE BLUE!

Having your picture in the paper or seeing yourself on TV is a joy, especially for something as noble as saving a life. Being in the public eye, emergency service workers are aware that they may appear in photos. So when someone notices media on scene, they do everything possible to look impressive, hoping to wind up on the six o'clock news or the front page.

Going back to my grade school days, I've had weird luck with the media. I went fishing for the first time when I was in the seventh grade— opening day of New Jersey trout season and I had no idea what I was doing. The river was stocked with fish, but the only things I managed to catch were a swan swimming across the river, my friend's father who was standing behind me – and a *massive* cold.

After standing in the freezing rain for several fruitless hours, we decided to pack it in. On the way back to the car, an elderly gentleman noticed we were empty-handed. Perhaps he was being generous, or maybe he was moved by how pathetic we looked. Whatever the reason, he offered us the dozen fish he had on a chain. We walked back to the car with the fish and caught the eye of a reporter. "Wow! You guys did great! Mind if I take your photo?" We said sure and posed. One of us was fishing, while the other two were admiring our "bountiful" catch. That photo made front page, dead center, and was used later for an annual fishing guide for the state.

My luck continued in emergency services. On one of the first big fires I was working on, I got chewed out by a chief for not being where I was supposed to me. A reporter took my photo for a national magazine and put a caption under it that read, "Firefighters discuss options at a large warehouse fire." Luckily the photo was from behind so no one could see the look of embarrassment on my face.

I had a streak where every photo of me in the local newspaper was from behind. People said they could recognize my butt anywhere.

During my first few months in Jersey City, I responded to a major motor vehicle accident. A drunk driver had run a stop sign and plowed into a mini van. The minivan, which was full, was thrown onto the sidewalk, running over several pedestrians. A news van from New York was on scene to capture the whole thing.

I was one of the last ambulances to get there, so I was given the drunk driver as a patient. I tried to examine him, but all he kept yelling about was his false teeth. They had been knocked out in the accident and he wanted to find them. I told him repeatedly not to worry about it since it was not on my list of priorities.

He continued to press on about his teeth. At one point he tried to climb off the backboard and get out of the ambulance. I grabbed him and threw him down on the board and yelled, "Nobody gives a fuck about your teeth, you drunk bastard! You nearly killed seven people, be thankful we don't kick your ass!"

I guess I should thank God for small favors. The *sound* of me yelling at him didn't come through on the news. But when my friends and family – and supervisors – turned on the eleven o'clock news, there I was yelling at my patient. Sure, they couldn't *hear* me, but they could *definitely* read my lips.

COPS was filming in Jersey City one summer and threw us into a frenzy; we were chomping at the bit to be on a call that would make a nationally syndicated TV show. Each night the topic of conversation was who saw cameramen on their jobs and whether it was interesting enough to make it on TV.

One evening I was dispatched to a suicidal man, sitting at the top of the steps in front of his house. He was crying and threatening to stab himself.

We entered right behind the police Emergency Services. They were decked out in their heavy ballistic vests and helmets as if they were making a tactical entry on a drug raid. It looked very impressive – extremely camera friendly. We began building a rapport with the patient, but he continued to threaten suicide. *COPS* was filming the whole thing. I kept thinking how great this would look on camera with me talking to a suicidal patient.

We were standing by as the police tried to talk him into putting down the knife. He was doing well until he noticed the camera. "I'm going to kill myself!"

"He's not going to kill himself," one of the officers told the cameramen, "keep rolling."

"I mean it! I'm going to do it."

The cameramen turned off the camera and started walking down the stairs. "Oh, well. Looks like he's going to do it," they said as they left the building. "We don't want to film that."

They won't film that, but they will film transvestite crack junkies getting mauled by a police dog when they try to run after an armed robbery?

COPS missed the chance to show a cool scene as the man's brother came and reduced the man to tears as he gently put his hand on the patient's shoulder and reassured him everything would be okay. When the man let his guard down, the Emergency Services pounced on him and subdued him. *That would have made for awesome TV.*

I did eventually manage to appear on *COPS* – and I managed to get acquitted (*Sorry, old joke. I know*).

We were dispatched for a hostage standoff in progress. We arrived just as Emergency Services were suited up for a tactical entry. It's always impressive to watch a SWAT team enter a building, so we stood by and watched.

My partner and I expected to be released after they found out it was a false alarm. But soon, a lady ran out of the building, escorted by an ESU officer. She was bawling her eyes out, and for some odd reason, that struck my partner as funny. "Hey, look at her. She looks upset."

We all had a chuckle, until we saw the camera behind her. "Oh shit, *COPS*!" I called out.

"Yeah, they're everywhere," my supervisor cracked.

"No, dude, the TV show!"

Suddenly we all froze and straightened up. So, I have been immortalized on *COPS* looking like the proverbial "deer caught in headlights."

The firehouse where I volunteered was doing another Fire Safety Week demonstration. The man running it was deaf. When he didn't have his hearing aids in, he tried to play if off by saying "Yeah. Yeah," to whatever you said.

The demonstration was widely publicized and drew the attention of New Jersey's biggest radio station, NJ101.5, who called and asked to speak to the man running things. We had no idea that the radio station was doing the interview live on the air. More importantly, we didn't know our man had forgotten his hearing aid.

"Hi, you're on the radio."

"Yeah." *Right away we started to hold our breath.*

"So we understand you're doing fire awareness doing there. What are you guys doing, lighting buildings on fire?"

"Yeah, yeah."

Our chief couldn't run fast enough to grab the phone away from him.

While on scene at a major fire, a friend of mine found that he needed to make some adjustments. Thinking no one was looking, he adjusted the crotch of his pants. That wasn't good enough, so he had to make a few more adjustments. Walking back to his truck, he received an urgent message on his pager to contact the chief *immediately.*

"Yeah, chief. What's up?"

There was dead silence on the phone as the chief composed himself. "Would you mind not playing with your balls on the nightly news!"

At that, he looked up and saw the local news helicopter hovering overhead. His adjustments had made the five o'clock and the six o'clock updates.

Standing by at a major warehouse fire, some co-workers and I started the Code Blue Game. The object is simple— try to look impressive so the cameras catch you. Then, when you are sure the cameras are on you, say stupid things to each other and see if you can read your lips on the news.

We found the best way to play Code Blue was to seek out the fire command post when the chief or public information officer is giving a briefing to the news cameras. Stand in the back of the shot and start pointing at the fire. Gesture with your hands to make it seem like you're pointing out important things to your partner. Then, say whatever you want. It works!

We were on scene at a four-alarm fire. The owner of the house where the fire started was being a complete pain in the neck. He had a right to be upset that his house burned down, but then he yelled at the firemen and EMTs who were first on the scene because he didn't think they got there fast enough. On top of that, he tried to go on the news and tell them the same thing. According to the taped radio transmissions, the first fire engine was on scene in less then three minutes, and in-service operating a hoseline two minutes after that. *Five minutes!* I guess he expected the fire department to be there before the fires start.

Having heard this, we got behind every news shot, making the official looking hand gestures and saying things like: "That rat bastard! How ungrateful!" "I'm glad your house burned down, you a-hole." We were also discussing our thoughts on the reporters who were on scene.

When we got back to headquarters to go home, someone stopped us. "Hey, I saw you guys on the news. Why were you calling that guy an 'a-hole?'"

On the way to my car, someone else stopped me. "Hey, Devin. What did you want to do to that hot reporter from *Telemundo?*"

HUDSON STREET AND
MONTGOMERY STREET

It's that time of the evening when all units available meet up at the local diner for dinner and gossip. I shake hands with the owner as I walk in. He smiles and yells my order back to the cook. We come here so often, he knows what we want before we do.

The back corner of the smoking section is filled with EMS uniforms. Being a non-smoker, I take a seat that appears to have the most fresh air. As soon as I sit down, the gossip starts – who's sleeping with whom, who's getting fired, who screwed up, etc. EMS can be a group of grown eight-year-olds. Apparently, our jobs aren't interesting enough so we have gossip about each other. Ten minutes into the conversation, another crew comes in and joins us. It's crew 315, and they're more smiley than usual. I think nothing of it and go about bullshitting.

I'm enjoying my cheeseburger and ice cold soda when I'm predictably interrupted. "309," the dispatcher calls over the radio, "I need you to respond to three forty five Gates Avenue, stage on Gates and Ocean, for the fire standby." All things considered, it could be worse. At least I'll get to sit around for a few minutes and eat my dinner while I'm on scene – providing there are no patients. My partner and I get up to leave. I wave a hand to everyone and start to walk out.

"Enjoy yourselves, guys," one of the crew of 315 calls out to us. I smile and nod, not quite understanding why he's so chipper.

Moments later we are barreling down Ocean Avenue towards the fire scene. Large crowds of people are congregating on Ocean, enjoying the warm summer evening. My partner takes his eyes off the road for a moment and looks between the seats. He quickly brings his attention back to the road. "Bro, do you smell something?" I take some exaggerated breaths but smell nothing. I shrug and shake my head. My partner shrugs and goes back to driving.

We are approaching the scene now. Two fire engines are lined up on the side of the road. My partner pulls over and calls to the dispatcher. I reach between the seats and grab my helmet. Then it hits me. There is a faint but rancid odor coming from somewhere in the truck. I hand my partner his helmet and we're about to step out to get the equipment when a fire chief approaches us. He politely informs us that we are cancelled and thanks us for coming out.

"Hey," I say to my partner, "I think I smell what you were talking about. What the heck is it?"

He leans his head back between the seats. A surprised look passes over his face. He turns down the stereo and leans back. "Do you hear something?"

I chuckle, "You're asking the wrong guy. I'm deaf in one ear."

My partner gets out and I follow. He opens up the rear doors and we immediately see the problem. "This is war!" My partner exclaims.

There, on our stretcher, with a pillow and a blanket to keep him warm with the air conditioner blasting on high, is one of our regular homeless patients.

"Jimmy!" I call to him, but he doesn't stir. I climb in and shake him on his shoulder. "Jimmy, get up!" He grumbles and rolls over. Laughing, I start forcefully rubbing my knuckle into his sternum.

"What the hell?" Jimmy yells as he fights my hand away.

"Jimmy, you can't sleep here."

"You're damn right I can't. Not with the way you two drive!"

Recovering from that comment, my partner says, "Jimmy, you gotta get out of the truck." Groggy from a day of sitting in the sun drinking, Jimmy tries to stand up, only to fall back onto the stretcher and begin snoring.

My partner shakes his head, climbs in, and puts the seat belts on Jimmy. "Come on," he says as he gets out. "City South Hospital is right around the corner. We'll go drop him off there."

EMS SUPERSTITIONS

After a while, most of us on the job tend to get a little superstitious. Some of us wear a lucky T-shirt under our uniforms or have lucky pens or things of that nature.

One superstition that seems to carry across squads throughout the country is feeding the pager. In diners across the country, you can see ambulance personnel seated at a table with sugar packets or French fries sitting on top of their pagers or radios. This is the only way to warn off the evil Call Gods while we eat. If the pager is appeased, no calls will come. If not, you'll never be able to finish your meal.

Then there are the ghosts. According to all the legends, ghosts are tortured spirits who haunt the place where they die because there is some sort of unfinished business. Thinking about all of the tortured people who have died and left unfinished business in the back of an ambulance, it's easy to see why many EMTs have had strange happenings in their trucks.

I had some eerie experiences in one particular ambulance. I knew the history of the truck when I got into it, but
I didn't believe any of it. Until...

Ambulance #44 had been dispatched to a life-
threatening call. As they pulled out to respond, a confused,
elderly woman stepped out in front of them and they hit
her. She died a few days later in intensive care. A few
months later, a different crew was dispatched in the same
truck for a cardiac arrest. As they were removing the patient
from the house, the patient's son blurted out, "Hey, isn't
this the truck that hit my mother a few months ago?" It was,
and the curse of #44 took affect.

Little poltergeist things started happening in the truck.
Electrical equipment would short out, equipment you
swore was there would be missing. Most of these things were
easily explained.

I was driving it one day and hit a small bump in the road.
The electrical equipment went out. I hit another small bump
and it came back on again. *Ok, that's easy enough to explain.*
Then I hit another bump and the equipment went out.
Another bump and it came back on. One more bump and
the entire truck stopped. I pulled over and checked the truck.
Diesel fuel and anti-freeze were pouring out of the bottom
and I had no electrical equipment working.

A tow truck brought the ambulance back. The
mechanics moved it inside the garage, which is attached to a
hospital. They popped the hood and tried to start it. Flames
began shooting out of the engine and lapping off the ceiling.
The brave mechanics ran out of the garage without hitting
the alarm to alert everyone in the hospital there was a fire in
the garage. *The sad part is that was the fastest I have ever
seen the mechanics move, and it was in the opposite
direction of where they were needed.* Seeing this, the chief
ran back in with a fire extinguisher. The mechanics followed

him, grabbing the garden hose we use to clean the trucks and put the fire out.

Several days later, the truck was ready and sitting by itself in our south station parking lot. I pulled into the station by myself and was backing my ambulance into a spot next to #44. As I pulled in next to it, #44's side door opened up and hit my ambulance. I thought someone was playing a trick on me but when I got out and checked the truck, no one was inside. No one was anywhere to be seen and my car was the only one in the parking lot. That was all I needed to see. I left the equipment where it was and got the heck out of there.

Like something out of a Stephen King novel, almost ten years to the day the elderly lady had been killed, the ambulance was broadsided by a truck while responding to a call. Finally totaled, #44 was taken out of service.

We had another ambulance that no one wanted to drive. This curse I can't explain. In the five years #24 was at work, it was only in service for about six months. Every time it went back into service, someone got into an accident with it.

Since I have been there, it was hit by two drunk drivers, ripped the bottom off against a high curb, and rolled over. The absolute best was the last time it was coming back from the shop. The flat bed it was on got into an accident and #24 rolled off the flat bed and overturned on the highway.

When it was finally ready to come back from that accident, our coordinator changed the number on the truck to #22 in hopes that it would avoid another accident for awhile. By now it was known affectionately as "The Pisser" because of all the urine tests the drivers had to take after they got into accidents.

Just to prove how sadistic we are (*or how* I *am*), I organized a pool on when the truck would crash again.

They had to match up the right two-week period with the right type of accident. The winner walked away a few weeks later with over $400 when someone broke a mirror on the truck.

We used to bet on one of our co-workers, one of the laziest people I had ever met. He would find any reason to go out of service. He once tried to go out of service to change his socks because it was during a heat wave and he was sweating. Of course, when he went out of service, we would all have to work harder. So rather than beat him senseless, we pooled on him: When would he go out of service, and for what reason?
I won $65. There was such a demand for a repeat that I tried to organize another pool. I was only able to collect $30 before he went out of service again.)

I don't believe in all the ghost stories I am told, but I firmly believe the building where I volunteer is haunted.
We have a rule that if you live within a certain distance from the building, you can respond to the building from home at night. Of course, I couldn't live within that distance, so I've spent many a night sleeping at the building alone.
I would lie on the couch late at night, and as soon as I turned off the TV, things would start happening. The door from the ambulance bay to the TV room would bang like someone just walked in. *Air conditioner just kicking in, okay.* Then I would hear footsteps leading from the ambulance bay, through the TV room to the bathroom. *Maybe it was the pipes. I'll buy that.* Then I would hear water running in the bathroom. *Maybe someone stopped by late at night.* Maybe, but maybe not. But no one was ever there.

After several months of this, I happen to run into one of the old founding members of the squad. He asked me how Anthony was doing.

"Who's Anthony?"

"Oh, he's the ghost in the building."

Oh, of course! How could I have not known? Nice of someone to tell me that those noises I heard at night had a name.

Then he told me the story. Back when the Squad first started, they held an annual awards dinner in the ambulance bay. Anthony, the squad's first captain was at a dinner one year. He left the ambulance bay to use the bathroom and died of a heart attack in the men's room.

I don't sound so crazy any more, do I?

A few people have tried to refute this, but I think it's all a conspiracy. We know the truth, and but it's not "out there." It's in the men's room.

PRACTICAL JOKES

Considering the stress level in the job that we do, it's a must that we somehow blow off steam - practical joke wars.

One of the standards is to mess with the door handles on the other person's ambulance. Lubricating jelly gives them that nice slippery feeling that's hard to wash off. Going the opposite end, oral glucose – sugar paste – gums up quickly and becomes very sticky and hard to wash off.

To counter one of these attacks and end the feud quickly, I usually place Nitroglycerin paste on the door handle. Nitro is used to dilate blood vessels in someone who's having a heart attack. One of the side effects is that it drops the blood pressure. So when you get it on your fingers, it usually drops the blood pressure enough to give you a killer headache and end the feud.

To end another feud, I took the clear plastic oxygen tubing and tied the front doors of the other ambulance together from the inside. When the crew came out to leave the hospital, they tried to open the doors, which yanked out of their hands and slammed shut.

A new member of my volunteer squad had an attitude problem that required some major adjustment. So after one call, we ganged up on him and tied him to a backboard. We inflated rubber gloves and taped them to his head so he looked like antlers. We then took photos of him and faxed them around the county.

I was asleep in the ambulance while my partner was getting something to eat. A homeless man started to hit him up for money. He told the homeless man to see me because I "handle finances for the ambulance tonight." The man would not leave me alone when I told him no and my partner just stood there and laughed.

We had a department picnic one summer. We had a ton of food, beer, and fun. To top if off, someone brought a pig to roast. We chopped the head off the pig and placed it in a new guy's ambulance without him knowing it. He was dispatched to a pedestrian struck soon after that. When he pulled out his stretcher in the middle of a crowded street, people began screaming at the sight of the pig's head sitting on his stretcher.

Several EMTs have personal pagers that give them updates of fires from around the area. This is all well and good, until they feel the need to announce that there is a five-alarm fire four states away. *Why do you need to know? Are you going to respond?*

A member at a friend's station was addicted to the pager. He would get up in the middle of the night to check the updates. The rest of the guys at the station managed to convince the operator from his paging service to page only him that there was a raging fire at his house.

Many squads use pagers that can only be set off by the dispatcher to alert them of a call. Some models save the last transmission so that you can repeat the dispatch in case you can't remember the address. I lucked out that the last dispatch on my pager was a working fire with possible people trapped. Around two in the morning after my new partner had just fallen asleep, I turned the sound up all the way, hit the repeat button, and watched him spring into action when he heard "working fire with entrapment." He was in the front seat of the ambulance and ready to go before I had the heart to tell him it was a joke.

My brother's friend got into an accident with the ambulance. While he was strapped down to the backboard in the Emergency Room, someone got a hold of his chart and scribbled "Warm Saline Enema" in hand writing pretty close to the doctor's.

A department was doing annual physicals for its employ-ees. One of the older, most homophobic members was getting a prostate exam. Another member crept in; and while the doctor had one hand on the man's shoulder and was using a finger of the other hand to exam the patient's prostate, he placed his hand on the other shoulder. The patient immediately tensed up and screamed.

One of the guys I worked with has problems staying awake after midnight. He fell asleep with a patient in the back on the way to the hospital. His partner arrived at the hospital, took the patient in, put the stretcher back in, slammed the door open and screamed, "Jesus Christ! Where the fuck's the patient?" His partner never fell asleep on a call after that.

When hanging out in a group, someone will inevitably say something stupid when someone else keys up the radio in hopes of having transmitted over the air. I'm guilty of finding this funny.

A group of us were talking when one of us was dispatched for "a man who can't see." My friend keyed up his radio to acknowledge the assignment and blurted out, "If he can't see, how the fuck did he dial the phone?"

After my friend was finished with that call, he had to try to explain it to management. Luckily, he didn't hang me out to dry and just played stupid.

Some coworkers rolled up on a scene for an assault. A large crowd of people was watching them get out of the truck. As one paramedic stepped out of the truck, his partner cranked up the radio and blasted Culture Club singing "I'll Tumble For You" so everyone could hear. The first medic's face lost all expression.

"What the hell are you doing?"

His partner looked at him with a serious face. "We're two white guys in the Projects listening to Culture Club... who's gonna mess with us?"

What worries me most here is where did they find a radio station that still plays that song?

I believe we are all big kids on this job. And boredom has the same results on us as on little kids. We start to play.

One Christmas Day things were slow. So my partner and I drove aimlessly around the city trying to find something to do. I pulled out some schoolbooks and studied while he drove. He pulled into a large unpaved lot, which was covered with a sheet of ice.

"Hey, what do you think will happen if we drove over that ice?" He asked me.

"I don't know. How deep do you think it is?"

"Oh, not deep at all." Famous last words. "Let's do it."

As we gunned the engine and prayed that somehow we could get free from the ice we had just sunk into, I couldn't help but laugh at how similar this was to a story in my first book. So I decided to use that solution to get us out of the hole we were stuck in. We grabbed some plastic backboards and tried to wedge them under the back wheels. What we didn't know was that the wooden backboards were what you were supposed to use. The plastic ones just slipped under the wheels and shot off far in front of the ambulance. We became very frantic, throwing tree branches and rocks and anything we could get our hands on under the wheels. Finally we gave up and called our supervisor and faced the music for fooling around.

Two years later, I went to interview for a promotion from EMT to Paramedic in the department. I sat down with the head of the department, and two of the other administrators. Everything was going great. The administration people and I were having a great time, laughing and joking, and I was knocking their "softball" questions out of the park.

The head of the department remained silent through the whole interview, only perusing my employee file. Everything was about to wrap up when the head of the department said, "I have just one question." *'One question' is never a good thing.* He slid out an incident report and I knew right away what it was. He studied it, twirled it around on the table for a moment, then cleared his throat. "So, you sank an ambulance?"

My heart sank, and the other administrators looked at me in horror.

"You don't plan on doing that to any of my medic trucks, do you?" he asked.

"No sir. Not at all."

He stared at me a moment longer – long enough for my heart to sink and my sphincter to tighten up – then smiled. "Lighten up."

On another quiet night, a crew was driving around and stumbled upon almost every kid's fantasy: construction equipment sitting behind a building, unlocked. It was midnight, and no one was around. (*So what else were they supposed to do?*) They hopped on and started playing with the bulldozers. They weren't destroying anything, just driving around the empty parking lot. They had the time of their lives. The supervisor didn't find it so amusing, watching their antics the next morning on the video from the store's security.

One night out of boredom, all the whackers on the shift took their blue lights out of their cars and put them on the ambulances. We turned off all the overhead lights and responded to jobs with the dashboard blue lights. Motorists were so surprised that they pulled over faster than they would have if we only used our overheads.

The all-time greatest practical joke I heard perpetrated (so far) was in response to a minor joke. A paramedic crew was taking a nap in the back of their truck. An EMT crew opened the doors and sprayed them with a water gun. *Not too original, but very effective when trying to piss someone off.*

In response, the paramedics took rolls of toilet paper and papered the EMTs' cars. What made it great was that it rained right after that, causing the paper to stick to the cars. The EMTs were stuck at work in the morning trying to get the paper off. Frustrated, one of them left a lot of it on the car and just drove home. On his way, his local police stopped him when they saw his vandalized car – adding insult to injury.

CITY SOUTH HOSPITAL ER

20:03 Hours

"Come Sunshine, time to get up," I pound on the side of the truck loudly to wake up Jimmy. He stirs, but doesn't get up. "Come on!" I climb in and give him a shake.

Getting frustrated, I bury my knuckles into his sternum and give him a hard rub. Predictably, he wakes up swinging. I catch his arm before he has a chance to connect. "Jimmy, sweetie," I plead, "don't be like that."

"Go to hell!" Suddenly, he's awake and trying to get off the stretcher.

My partner climbs inside and takes a hold of Jimmy's other arm. "Enough fooling around. Let's go!"

"I'm not going," he protests. Jimmy puts up a hell of a fight but we manage to pull him to his feet. I catch a glimpse of large wet spot on the stretcher. Surrounding it are brown streaks that I pray are just dirt from him lying on the ground.

Jimmy stumbles on his way out. My partner catches him falling out of the truck. "Oh god, Jimmy! Ain't you ever heard of a shower?"

"Shut up!" He slurs angrily. "I'll kick your ass." I catch a whiff of the alcohol and decay in his mouth and I shutter to think about what my partner smells being face to face with the guy.

We carry Jimmy into the waiting room, his feet dragging behind us as he tries to fight us. We place him in a chair as far away from other people as we can. "Ma'am," I say to the elderly women nearest to him, "I apologize for the smell." She gives me an uneasy smile.

"Come back here and fight like a man!" Jimmy yells to me. "I'll kick your fucking asses!"

"Jimmy," my partner admonishes him, "watch your mouth! There are women and children here."

"I'll kick your ass!" Jimmy stands up and squares off in an unsteady fight stance.

"Jimmy, sit down."

"You a chicken?" Jimmy pumps his fists towards my partner.

My partner looks around at the inquiring eyes of the people in the waiting room. I know my partner would like nothing better than to knock this guy out, but Jimmy really isn't worth getting fired over. Instead, my partner laughs in his face. "Jimmy, please."

Jimmy takes a swing at my partner. My partner simply shifts to the side and watches as Jimmy falls to the ground. "Come on, Sunshine," I say as I lift him off the ground, "You just bought yourself four-point restraints."

He weakly protests as we carry him into the ER. "You guys know Jimmy?" My partner asks as we walk into the back. We deposit Jimmy on a bed and assist security in placing him in leather restraints.

I sit down at the desk and start filling out my paperwork. I would have dumped him in the waiting room and let him sleep off the alcohol had he not tried to fight. "Those bastards!" I look over and see my partner looking out the window at the ambulance parking lot.

The crew of 315 is parked outside. Both members are standing outside and laughing at our truck. "Oh, it's on!" I help myself to the medication cabinet in the ER. *A little Calcium Chloride and Dextrose should do the trick...*

Without saying a word, I walk past 315 to their truck with the tubes of medication. "Hey, Devin," one of them asks, "what are you doing?" I take the meds, mix them together and spray them all over the windshield. They cake up into a hard white crust that I know will be a pain in the ass to clean off.

"Game's over," I say nonchalantly as I get back in my truck.

Payback's definitely a bitch...

THE PARTNER FROM HELL

It's horrible to work with a bad partner. I've had my share of them over the past couple of years, but one stands out in my mind. He's not really a bad person, but one day he drove me up the wall.

It started off okay. I came in for my night shift after being at school all day, picked up my equipment and checked the schedule to see whom I was working with. A shudder ran down my back as I read the roster. I'd worked with this guy a week or two before and didn't have a problem, but I had a gut instinct that this would not be a good night.

We had our first job about a half-hour into the shift— a call for a stabbing on the outside of one of the city's housing projects. My adrenaline got pumping as I sped to the call. Dodging cars and pedestrians, I turned the radio up so I could have some driving music. He immediately turned down the radio. *Big mistake! You don't mess with the radio when you're the passenger.* Then he cranked up the heat in the truck. Sure it was cold, but the hairs on my legs felt like they were going to spontaneously ignite. *Another big mistake! The driver has the final say in the climate control of the vehicle.*

We pulled up on scene and were told by the police that the call was unfounded. They had checked the area and were satisfied that someone had made a phony 911 call.

En route to our post area, I heard on the radio that another unit had happened upon an accident and needed assistance. It was in our area so I volunteered for the call. "Why did you do that?" he asked me, sounding very annoyed.

"Because it's in our area."

"You don't take a job without asking your partner. Didn't anyone ever tell you that?"

I bit my tongue, said nothing, and headed for the accident. In a way, I was glad I took the call. In the middle of a busy street, there was an accident involving a station wagon, a mini-van, and a boat. Yes, that's right. Sitting on top of this twisted wreckage was a boat. The story came out later that a drunk driver and his friend were driving the station wagon, coming back from a long day of drinking and fishing (hence the boat). They misjudged a turn and wrapped themselves around the van. The boat came loose and went through the back window of the station wagon and gave the driver a depressed skull fracture. *Pretty cool, right?*

Our patients were from the van. They weren't hurt that bad, but the driver required a backboard. We must have been on scene for at least twenty minutes while we sorted through the mess with our chief, getting stories, assessing patients, and packaging. After ten minutes I got antsy and wanted to move to the hospital; it's just the way I am. So I packaged my patient and stepped out to drive. "Ah, aren't you going to check his blood pressure?" I was taken back at first by his rude tone.

"You can't do it while I drive to the hospital?"

"Ah, no. I have paperwork to do."

I decided to play along with this for now. I took a few deep breaths (*Out with the bad, in with the good.*), and stepped back in. I checked the blood pressure and drove to the hospital.

After putting the truck back in order, our dispatcher asked us if we could handle a call. We had been at the hospital longer than the ten minutes we're generally allotted for paperwork and clean up, and I knew we were the only ambulance available, so I said sure. He came flying out of the ER, screaming at me for taking the call. "You should always consult with me first. I'm not done with my paperwork! This is bullshit!"

"Why didn't you do it while we were driving to the hospital?"

"Because I can't write with the way you drive."

Now I happen to think I'm a good driver. "Then you could have checked the blood pressure," I said as I climbed in the driver's seat and let the sound of the diesel engine and the radio drown him out. We were sent literally around the corner for an assault.

As I pulled up, I saw a few police officers standing by a young man seated on the curb. The young man was holding his head and had a look of pain of his face. We stepped out of the truck and approached him. "Sir, what's the problem?" I took out my flashlight and went to examine him.

"That guy hit me in the back of the head with a shovel."

Without even looking at the patient, my partner pipes up very condescendingly, "Oh yeah, I can really see the dent!" He was right in a way; there was no dent. However, there was a huge lump on the back of his head.

"Look, you go inside and check on the other guy," I ordered him. He left in a huff and went inside to check on another patient the police found inside. I tried my best to convince him to go to the hospital, but the patient was so annoyed with my partner that he wanted nothing to do with us. So, begrudgingly, I had him sign the refusal. The patient inside the house also signed a refusal, and with that we were back in service.

Next we were dispatched for one of our regulars. He always hung out outside of a Post Office with his boys. He acted differently to different EMTs. If you treated him like a human being, more often than not he's civil to you. If you treat him with disrespect, like we are often tempted to do because he calls the ambulance *at least* once a day, then you'll have problems with him. I'm usually nice to him, regardless of how many times I pick him up, because I like to practice confrontation avoidance. I had been picking him up for four years and knew he was an alcoholic, but I had no idea he was asthmatic.

This time I found him in the tripod position—a tip-off that the patient is in severe respiratory distress. He could barely say that he was having trouble breathing. I listened to his lungs and heard nasty congestion and some asthma wheezing. The wheezing wasn't that bad, but the congestion concerned me because I knew he was homeless and at great risk for pneumonia.

"Maybe if you didn't drink so much this wouldn't happen to you."

I dropped my stethoscope and turned to him, "What the hell did you just say?"

My partner looked at me with a grin on his face. "I said if he didn't drink so much, we wouldn't be here to pick him up."

"Are you paying attention to anything that's going on?"

"Yeah, he's drunk again."

Blaming his drinking for his calls because he fell down or has a headache is one thing. However, I may be going out on a limb with this one, I can say with some certainty that his drinking *probably* had nothing to do with his developing pneumonia. *Call me crazy, but that's my thinking.* Think my partner would have a little more sympathy for the man being that he is also a bad asthmatic? Of course not!

After quieting down my patient because he wanted to rip my partner's head off, and I was thinking of letting him, we were en route to the hospital.

For our next call we raced across town next for a baby with a fever. Right away I knew this was going to be an unpleasant experience. No one in the house spoke English, except for the baby's 13 year-old aunt, and there was a drunken old man in the corner yelling at us in Spanish. From what I could piece together with my limited knowledge of Spanish, he was pissed off that it had taken us three hours to get there. I knew and he knew it didn't take us that long to get there, but I wasn't about to argue with him. I made a command decision to scoop up the baby and do the assessment in the safety of the ambulance en route to the hospital.

But it couldn't be that simple. My partner wanted to stay and assess the patient in the room. That might not have been so bad if there wasn't the belligerent drunk in the kitchen next to the knives. And I'm sure I probably would have let him continue the assessment if he had tried talking to the only English speaking person in the room instead of ignoring the young girl. So, much to his dismay, I grabbed the child and hurried everyone out of the apartment to the ambulance. The baby appeared fine and in no distress, so my usual course of action is load up the parents, get going to the hospital, and do the assessment en route. As I tried to put the ambulance in drive, he yelled at me. "I need to take a blood pressure first!"

Normally, I would have yelled right back at him. But seeing as the baby was only a few months old and I knew we didn't have a blood pressure cuff that small, this I had to see.

After a few minutes of him struggling, I just left and went to the hospital.

After that we were dispatched to the South District Police Station for a sick prisoner. I decided I would take Kennedy Boulevard all the way south because it offered four lanes of traffic as opposed to going down Bergen Ave (where the police station is) which has only two lanes and is chronically congested with double-parked cars. "Oh, did you forget how to get to the South District?"

"Look, if you can do a better job driving, by all means do it!" Of course, I wasn't about to surrender the keys to him.

Mercifully, we were cancelled from that assignment.

After that, we stopped by headquarters and I was complaining to the chief about him. Somehow I slipped up somewhere and my partner got a hold of the keys. *Big mistake on my part!*

I didn't have the energy to argue, so I just got in the passenger seat and let him drive. *How bad could it possibly be?* I would find out.

We were driving around aimlessly when I heard a call go out for a violent, emotionally disturbed person on Gardner Ave, a few blocks from where we were. I thought about taking it, but then decided the less the amount of calls I go on with him the better. But as we were passing Gardner Ave, he saw a group of kids walking across the street laughing. Granted, it was two in the morning and they were *probably* up to no good, but all they were doing was walking across the street. So he panics, and shoots the wrong way up Gardner Ave and right past the police officers in front of the house.

A few minutes later, the dispatcher called the unit that was dispatched to that location and told them the police called and said they missed the house. I felt bad because I didn't want the other truck to get in trouble. So I went to call on the radio to tell them we drove past the house and offer to take the call, as we were right there anyway. He slapped the radio out of my hand!

At this point, my island of calm and rationality could feel an angry tidal wave coming on.

We were dispatched for a pregnant lady in labor. We arrived and knocked on her door for a few minutes. Finally, we were able to wake up her neighbor downstairs. Our patient was upstairs getting ready to go and didn't hear us knocking. No big deal. I was glad she wasn't in need of *immediate* attention.

We asked a few preliminary questions and I set up the stair chair. She took one look at that and said, "Oh, you are *not* going to carry me downstairs on that! I'll walk."

That was all I needed to hear. I put the chair away and offered her my arm to hold onto while we walked downstairs. I'm not lazy, but if she thinks she can walk I'm not going to stop her.

Things were running smoothly. She was walking, my partner hadn't said anything, and life was good for a moment. Then, things changed, and he felt the need to speak up. "Come on, ma'am. Let's move."

"I'm walking as fast as I can."

"Didn't anyone ever tell you walking is good for you?"

"Didn't anyone ever tell you that you're an asshole?" *Thank you, ma'am! Couldn't have said it better myself.*

I helped her into the ambulance and sat her on the stretcher. "Oh, she doesn't need to go on that."

"What are you saying? Just drive the truck!"

"No. I have to get a blood pressure."

"I'll do it en route, just drive."

"No. I have to get it now."

The patient began to yell at him between contractions. "Let him do it on the way! Just get me there. This hurts!"

"Hey lady, pain is part of being pregnant!"

Luckily for him, she was in too much pain to get up and

rip his head off. "What the fuck do you know about being pregnant?"

"I have a daughter."

"So? Did you carry her? Do you have a uterus? What the fuck do you know about being pregnant?"

He was about to say something to her, but I grabbed him by the arm and pushed him out of the truck.

When we got to the hospital, I saw a man standing outside of the ER entrance. He was trying to steady himself against the wall and trying to push the button to get someone to let him into the ER. From twenty feet away I could tell he was having trouble breathing. After a while an EMT is able to spot someone who's going to have to be intubated, and he was one.

"Sir, what's wrong?" I called as I pulled the stretcher out.

He mouthed the word 'asthma' to me. As I got closer, I couldn't hear any sound coming from him when he struggled to breathe. *Not a good sign at all!* I told my partner to take the patient upstairs to Labor and Delivery while I helped this guy inside.

"Oh, he's not our problem. Let security take him!"

"No! Obviously security isn't going to help him, and he'll die if I don't."

"But..."

"No buts, just take her upstairs!" I helped the man inside onto a chair just inside the door. Then I ran down the hall and grabbed a stretcher. As soon as I wheeled him into the Trauma Room, the doctor intubated him.

I went upstairs fuming and lost it when I walked into the L&D room. The patient and my partner were yelling at each other. Embarrassed beyond belief, I grabbed my partner and pushed him out of the room. Then I attempted to apologize to the patient as I helped her onto her bed. However, she wanted to hear none of that and dismissed me.

I can't say that I blame her. I wouldn't want to talk to us after the way my partner talked to her.

"Why are you being so nice to her? She's a loser!"

"What? Why couldn't you have just been nice to her?"

As if the entire night didn't just happen, he had the nerve to ask, "What's your problem?"

"What's my problem? You *are* an asshole, and you've *been* an asshole to every one of our patients tonight."

"I have not!"

I guess I was paying attention to another partner all night.

Yeah, there's nothing worse than being stuck with a horrible partner for 12 hours. I have been stuck with other bad partners, too. One didn't talk to me the entire shift. Another complained about my driving until finally I let her drive, and she crashed.

As much as I complain though, here is one co-worker I feel sorry for. She's been working in the department for several years and had the misfortune of being stuck with one of the newest employees. They were dispatched to a housing project for a confirmed stabbing.

They rolled up on scene and the police were swarming all over the complex. There was a large crowd of people yelling at the police, but it was safe to say that the scene was pretty well secured. She stepped off the truck, grabbed the jump bag and some supplies and ran into the building.

Her partner walked up to the first police officer he saw and asked how he would get to the trauma center from here. The officer told him where to go and walked off to handle some part of the investigation. Her partner grabbed his personal belongings and started walking for the main street. He got on the right bus and headed back to headquarters. He walked into the coordinator's office and turned in his equipment and went home, leaving his partner was stuck on the scene alone. She had to get a police officer to drive the ambulance.

Needless to say, he has never shown his face in the city again - *probably the first wise decision he's ever made!*

Being a brand new medic and the low man on the seniority totem pole, I got stuck working with many partners no one else wanted. I always smiled and said that I didn't mind because I was new and wanted to experience as much as possible. That notion didn't last long.

One partner I had to work with every other week drove me insane! The man would not shut up from the beginning of the shift till the end. To make matters worse, he would never talk about anything I wanted to talk about. I must admit, on the plus side, I became a lot better at completely blocking someone out.

Working on a call with him was like watching *COPS* – and anyone who's been on an ambulance has probably worked with someone like this. Just out of nowhere he would start giving a blow by blow of the call – as if I were paying attention to another call.

On top of all that, he would drive at 26 mph to a call. I could fall asleep on the way to a call and wake up feeling refreshed by the time we got there. Once we arrived just as the ambulance was pulling away. I called them on the radio and asked if the ambulance crew wanted to pull over so we could treat the patient. They said no, then raced to the hospital that was only a few blocks away anyway. My partner drove back to their dispatcher and yelled at her. "I'm not going to kill myself to get to these calls if your ambulance is going to pull away without us!"

Twenty-six mph is killing yourself?

A friend was dispatched as the first-in ambulance for a train derailment with 700+ patients. On the way to the job, his partner lost control of the ambulance and wiped out. Both were trapped in the ambulance and required extrication (as if the system wasn't already taxed with 700 patients). He was badly injured. He had fractured his femur and collapsed a lung on top of everything else. His injuries were so bad that paramedics had to decompress his chest.

While visiting him in the hospital, a co-worker offered his condolences. "Hey man, I'm sorry we had to pop your chest. You must be going insane cooped up here."

"Are you kidding? Can you imagine working a train derailment with *my partner*?"

I realize I'm awfully quick to criticize. I can be a real pain in the ass if I want to be. I don't believe in being fake and pretending to like someone. That takes entirely too much energy. If I don't like you, either I won't say anything to you or I'll try to make you cry.

I had to work with someone who always rubbed me the wrong way. I had heard how he drove the other people I like nuts, so that was a strike against him. Then I would hear him on the radio jumping every call possible. I'm not lazy, but I'll have none of that. I don't like to work that hard unless it's absolutely necessary.

Within the first few minutes of the shift he managed to piss me off. When I arrived, I found him sitting in the driver's seat. I don't mind sharing driving responsibilities with anyone, but if you just got hired don't try to assume that I'll let you drive. A group of co-workers were outside at shift change and witnessed this. They began teasing me about it, and I hate to be teased. "Watch this," I said as I walked over to the truck.

"Oh, I'm working with you?" I asked. "Good, give me the keys."

The look on his face was priceless. He looked like I had just killed his brother. "But I'm driving first half."

"Oh, I'm sorry. Maybe I mumbled. Give me the keys."

In front of everyone he got out of the driver's seat and stormed off inside. Everyone burst into laughter as he walked away. A few minutes later, a friend came out and told me that my partner was asking people to switch with him so he wouldn't have to work with me. *And we hadn't even done one call yet!*

No one would switch with him, so now it was fun time. We were dispatched to stand by at a working fire. Three minutes go by and he's not even outside yet. So I walk back inside and found him talking on the phone in the crew room. "You know we got a job, right?"

"Yeah."

"Oh, okay." Then raising my voice sharply, "Well, do you want to join me sometime today, new guy!" He jumped and dropped the phone. For the rest of the day I said nothing to him that wasn't absolutely necessary, and I tortured him by making him listen to talk radio and heavy metal music all day.

I know I can be a prick sometimes.

6TH STREET

20:15 hours

No rest for the weary!

I'm sitting in the passenger seat scanning the area for a "sick person – unknown complaint." I call on the radio and ask my dispatcher if she has any more information about where I might find my patient. Just as I finish my question, a heavy-set lady runs into the street waving her arms frantically. I instinctively slam my foot down on the floor, hoping to activate some imaginary brake. My partner gasps and practically stands up on the real brake pedal in a desperate effort to avoid hitting the lady.

We take a moment to catch our breath and check our underwear for any slippage induced by the shock of almost running someone over. She doesn't wait for us to get out of the ambulance. She is at the driver's side window, slapping her hands against it and yelling rapidly in Spanish.

With my amazing mastery of the Spanish language, I have absolutely no idea what she is saying. Luckily, my partner speaks a little Spanish. We follow the lady, straining to keep up with her run, and find a disheveled man slumped over on a doorstep. There is another man standing over him with a cordless house telephone in his hand.

"What's going on here?" I ask. The man responds by yammering away in Spanish. I hold my hands to halt him. "Do you speak English?"

"Yes."

"Then why don't we try talking in English?" My Spanish only allows me to ask where the bathroom is and to tell someone I don't speak Spanish – and even those I think I get wrong.

The man with the phone tells me this guy on his doorstep stumbled there, yelling something about his sore feet. I look at the man on the step and see that he is rocking himself back and forth, clutching his right leg. As I get closer, I catch a whiff of that odor I like to call *decaying human*. It is mixed with a heavy dose of rum and urine, making for an almost immediate wretch.

Above his shoe, I notice the end of an Ace bandage dangling down. I put on a pair of gloves and slide the pant leg up. It only takes a second for me to register the festering boils showing above the bandage. There is a new smell added to the mix. It's the sour milk smell of decaying flesh. My stomach tightens and I can feel my juices making their way up my esophagus. I drop the pant leg and spring back like I just discovered a bomb.

My partner, bewildered by my reaction, slips on a glove and slides up the pant leg. He has the exact reaction I have. Bracing ourselves for an impending bout of vomiting, we support the man under his arms and guide him over to the ambulance. Once inside, my first course of action is to turn on the vent fan and crank up the air conditioner.

My partner pats down the man for a wallet and hands me the man's ID. Gagging, my partner hurries to the front of the ambulance and starts to head out for the hospital.

The man continually tries to lie down on the bench seat. Each time I tell him to remain seated while the ambulance is moving. I don't know if he's purposely trying to piss me off or if he thinks I didn't get quite a good look at the catastrophe that is his leg, but he slides his pant leg up to his knee and exposes his wound once again. I yell for him to stop, but it is too late. Bare, rotten flesh has come in contact with my bench seat. My Funk-O-Meter goes off the scale, and I silently curse him for rendering that bench seat unusable for a nap later.

My partner opens the side door when we arrive at the ER entrance for Christ Our Savior Hospital. He laughs as he finds me with my undershirt covering my mouth and my head near the AC struggling for fresh air. "Burn that seat, please," I plead to him as we walk our patient inside.

The nurses inside are less than jovial to see us – I imagine it's been a rough day for them too. "What did you bring me?" The charge nurse asks after giving our patient a swift glance. "Another drunk?"

"I wish that was his real problem."

She gives me a cynical look, so I use my still gloved hand to expose his leg yet again. With each time it gets a little easier to handle. Soon, I am positive I will view it with twisted fascination. The nurse gasps. "Oh my god! Put him in bed ten!"

The pretty nurse handling bed ten gives my partner and I a flirtatious smile. She is about to give me a hug when she sees our patient slumped between to two of us. "Damn it! Are no other hospitals open tonight?"

Thanks friend! You ruined my bench seat and there goes my hug!

"What is that smell?" She asks.

My partner nods to our patient.

"You know," I offer, "I did a science experiment in the seventh grade in which I left a petri dish full of milk out on the window sill for an entire summer just to see what would happen. When I went back to school in the fall it smelled a lot like him."

The nurse looks at me in wonder, "They let you do that?"

"Well, not exactly. They didn't know it was me. What they don't know won't fail me."

We assist the man onto the bed. Curious family members of other patients are looking in on our patient. Seeing this, my partner announces rather loudly, "Devin, I'll bet you twenty bucks there's maggots under that wrapping." The once curious people look away in disgust.

It's a good thing I'm not a betting man. When the nurse unwraps the Ace bandage, several small, yellow maggots fall to the ground. I look on, unable to avert my eyes. From his kneecap down looks like it had suffered third degree burns. Several layers of skin appear to have been eaten away, exposing muscle and fatty tissue in some areas. The stench is overpowering and I leave the room dry heaving.

"Nurse!" The man in the next bed calls out. "I want you to switch my bed now!"

I dump generous amounts of alcohol on my bench seat in a desperate attempt to erase the memory of what was just sitting there. My mind flashes back to the sight of that waxy, bloated leg exposed on my seat. Then, I see the maggots falling out of his dressing.

My partner comes out of the ER with a smile on his face. "Hey, I wonder what else he had growing on him!"

That's all I needed to hear. Suddenly, it happens.

I feel it first on the side of my head, just above my ear. It seems harmless enough at first. Then I feel it between my shoulder blades and all up and down my arms. I suddenly itch all over thinking about bugs crawling on him, and making happy little homes on my bench. I frantically scratch my head. When I've managed to compose myself, I dump an entire bottle of alcohol on to the bench – contemplating briefly lighting it on fire.

They really do not pay me enough for this. It doesn't matter much now anyway. I think I left my appetite back at the scene.

GETTING DOWN AND DIRTY

Stories about feces and bugs are always good for shock value. As much as we would all like to believe that all of our calls are nice and clean like on *Rescue 911*, the truth is much nastier.

I responded for an elderly lady in respiratory distress. I arrived to find a sad sight. The lady was ravaged by cancer. The pictures of her on the wall looked nothing like the shape before me. She said she couldn't breathe. She began coughing and a large, bright red clump came out. I turned to my partner and said, "Scott, you better let the paramedics know she's throwing up large blood clots."

"Oh, that's not a blood clot," the husband said as he rushed into the room. "That's not a blood clot."

"Then what is it?"

"That's just liquid Tylenol."

"Sir, it's bright red and has the consistency of blood."

Then, to my disgust, he picked the clump off the floor and started running it through his hands. "See, it doesn't have the consistency of blood, it's a little thicker." He held it out to me as if offering it for my inspection.

When I didn't take it, he drew it back and started sniffing it. "It doesn't smell like blood." Finally, as if that wasn't bad enough, he dipped his finger in it, then tasted his finger. "See, cherry flavored!"

I don't care if that was cherry Tylenol, and I don't care if that was your wife of fifty years. You don't taste test something that was just expelled from someone's body.

I responded for a young child who was sick. The mother met us at the door with a zip lock bag in her hands. I couldn't see what was in it, and therefore didn't pay any attention to it. I just walked upstairs and began to examine the child.

The mother told me that her son was complaining of abdominal pains and had worms in his stool. If that wasn't bad enough, she wanted to know if I wanted to see. "No, that's not necessary," I replied.

"Yes it is! Here!" She thrust the zip lock bag in front of my face. Inside was a large pile of crap with what appeared to be worms in it. The smell hit me and I nearly passed out.

But the fun didn't stop there. Oh no! She tells me *I* have to carry the bag downstairs. I told her "Absolutely not. Your son produced it. He's your responsibility. You carry it." Would you believe she actually got mad at me for that?

"I don't want to carry it!" she yelled at me. *Too bad! One of my cardinal rules of patient care: if the patient produced it, the patient enjoys it! As you're the legal guardian, you get to enjoy it.*

Some of the weirdest things can be witnessed just by keeping your eyes open as you drive around. It was a very hot summer night, around 8 PM. I was driving through an area of Jersey City where a lot of people hang out during the summer. It was still bright outside and I was watching for any children running across the street.

"Damn it." My partner said. "Let's get out of here before we have to help that lady over there."

"What lady?"

"The one on the corner over there throwing up next to that guy." He pointed out a lady on knees right on the corner of a busy intersection. I instinctively stopped the ambulance to get a better look.

"Bro, she ain't throwing up." I said. "At least not yet." With that, my partner gave another look and realized…she was giving the man oral sex. *Right on the frigging street corner!*

I was driving around Jersey City in between calls. A nice day in early May, the sun was shining, the kids were out playing, and the Wandering Crapper was on the prowl.

The Wandering Crapper is not usually a problem. He walks around the streets picking up discarded cigarette butts and smoking what's left of them. Every now and then I see him digging through someone's garbage for something to eat. He's not usually a problem for society, and he never calls the ambulance for stupid reasons. *That's a plus in my book!*

So why do we call him the Wandering Crapper? That's because he is constantly wondering around, and he always shits on himself. On this particular occasion, we were driving along when my partner yelled to me, "That is absolutely disgusting!"

I looked over and saw the Crapper walking in front of a school playground, with his pants around his ankles. "You know," I said to my partner, "I really hate to get involved, but I think we kinda have to now."

We got out and approached him. He was friendly enough, as he usually is. We began trying to talk him into going to the hospital, positioning ourselves to shield the children from this man's nakedness. You may be asking why we talked him into going to the hospital if he wasn't complaining of anything. It was either that or he gets locked up for indecent exposure, and I didn't want to see that happen. *See, I can be a nice guy sometimes.*

We started to walk him towards the ambulance when he tripped over his pants. "I guess we should pull those up," I said with a sigh. My partner and I flipped a coin for it, and you shouldn't even have to guess who lost. As I bent down to pick up his pants, I heard an almost silent flutter of air which alarmed me just in time to dodge the crap as it fell out of his ass.

I feel bad for the Wandering Crapper. Not just because he has psychiatric problems, and not just because he lives in a boarding housee that I wouldn't wish upon my worst enemy, but because I feel slightly responsible for hospitaliz-ing him one night. Before all of the personal injury attorneys start combing the city for a man walking around with his pants around his ankles and crap falling, it wasn't completely my fault. It might not have even had anything to do with me, but what a coincidence!

I love a particular fried chicken restaurant. One evening I decided to try a hotter hot sauce than usual on my wings. As usual I got a call in the middle of dinner. Another and another and another followed that, so by the time I got to finish my dinner the grease had congealed. My stomach turned at the sight of all that grease and hot sauce, so I tossed the carton on top of some empty cardboard boxes. How was I supposed to know that the Wandering Crapper would pick *that* night to dig through the dumpster near the EMS garage? Someone saw him pull out a Styrofoam container and just let him be. A couple of hours later he was in the emergency room complaining of severe abdomi-nal pains and diarrhea. He told the nurse, "It must have been something I ate."

I was dispatched for a man lying in the street, in the snow, not moving one New Year's Eve. We drove up and down the street and found nothing. I was about to call back in service when one of the police officers found our patient. *Gee, thanks!*

He was hiding under the porch to a house, lying in about two to three feet of snow. It was dark, so I didn't get a chance to get a good look at him before I heard the officer say, "For Christ's sakes man, put your damn pants back on! It's freezing out here!"

The police officers recognized almost immediately that the man was on some type of controlled substance. Their suspicions were confirmed when a "friend" came out of the house to tell us that the man had been using Dip that night.

A combination of marijuana, formaldehyde and/or PCP, Dip is a weird drug. *Why anyone would smoke embalming fluid is beyond me.* But Dip will either make you extremely violent, or a totally mindless zombie. However, the zombie patient can easily go into a violent outrage at the drop of a hat. So we always take personal safety seriously when faced with Dip.

The police began trying their best to calmly talk the man into coming out and going to the hospital. Finally, as more officers arrived and the cold became unbearable, they decided to grab him and force him into the ambulance. They moved so fast that they literally scared the shit out of him, *and all over my bus!* They picked him up by his legs and arms and carried him into the ambulance, where they sat him on the bench seat and he smeared feces on it as they did so. Then they handcuffed him to the stretcher, making sure that the fun got spread all around.

At this, the man began screaming like a banshee. Luckily for me, I'm going deaf, so his high-pitched, bloodcurdling screams didn't phase me. They did, however, carry over the radio as I keyed up to call the dispatcher. So when I arrived at the hospital, all of my co-workers were there to great me and ask, "What are you guys doing to her?"

"Her? That ain't no her?"

They all stood in amazement as I wheeled this strong, muscle bound man out of the ambulance as he was screaming. I brought him into the ER and the doctor's first question without looking at the patient was "What's wrong with her?"

A lady suffering from severe postpartum depression decided to end it all. She jumped off the roof of her six-story New York City apartment building. The EMS and emergency room staff worked feverishly to save her. However, every time they compressed her chest, milk would shoot out of her breasts and hit one of the rescuers.

An ambulance responded to a housing project in Jersey City for a sick person. When they reached the apartment, they found a young girl playing in the living room and her sick mother in the bedroom. As they interviewed the mother, they could hear the child talking to herself in the other room. She appeared to be playing with some small toys and having a grand old time.

The mother got ready to go to the hospital and told the child she had to "put her friends away now." Curious, the crew went over to see what the girl was playing with.

To their shock and disgust, the girl had a box full of live cockroaches. She said that she kept them as pets. On the backs of each little, disgusting bug, was a design in nail polish. She said that she could tell the roaches apart by the design and they all had names. *There has to be a better way of entertaining yourself.*

I went to a family's house for a child crying. *Yes, that was the call.* The house was a disgrace. Garbage was strewn all over, as were beer cans. There was a funky moldy smell in the air, like the house had not had a good cleaning in years.

Being allergic to cats, I can almost tell right away when I walk into the house that there is a cat in the room. I got that feeling, looked around, and sure enough a fat cat was staring at me from the corner of the room. I found it odd that the cat was able to eat so well when everyone else in the house was skinny. Then I saw why. The cat was busying himself with eating out of his bowl when a cockroach climbed in. The cat immediately gobbled up the roach. I stood dumbfounded. Then another roach met the same fate and I nearly passed out. *Kinda makes you wonder what the rest of the house is dining on.*

I responded to a senior citizens' complex for a fall victim. The couple was the sweetest couple I have ever met. If I had a choice in how I would grow old, I would definitely want to age like them. But I sure as hell wouldn't want to live in the same place.

I was interviewing the patient while my partner was checking the lady's blood pressure. We were all laughing and joking. Then I looked down at my clipboard and saw a cockroach scampering across it. I quickly flicked it off. Recomposing myself with a few deep breaths, I went on talking like nothing happened. No one noticed anything was wrong.

I was just about finished with my interview when I looked down and saw another roach on the clipboard. Now I began to really feel skeevy and nauseous. I began to frantically swipe at the bug with a piece of paper. It wouldn't come off—just kept running around. No one in the room noticed me because my partner had everyone's attention. In a last ditch effort, I flicked it off. The bug soared through the air and hit the husband in the forehead. It ricocheted off his head and landed down the patient's dress. Still, somehow, no one noticed.

It was an uncomfortable ride to the hospital. Every now and then, the patient would scratch at her chest. I think I held my breath the whole way, waiting for the cockroach to pop up for a visit. *Thank goodness it didn't. I do believe I would have hurled if I saw it again.*

Ah, what the Hell! One more cockroach story for the road!

I responded to a welfare motel for an elderly lady who had fallen. When we arrived, she was lying face down on the floor next to her bed. She was moaning, so I knew she was alive. My partner and I knelt down next to her and got ready to move her. When we rolled her over, roaches came scurrying out of the pocket of her shirt and from her mouth. I felt pretty queasy, but my partner looked down and let out a bloodcurdling scream as she dove out of the apartment.

An ambulance responded for a sick person call in Trenton, NJ. As the crew approached the front door, they could smell a putrid mix of human excrement, rotten meat, and garbage. The scene inside was even worse. Garbage was thrown around the house, rats and bugs ran freely across the floor, and at various intervals throughout the house there were piles of shit.

Um, I can't be sure, but I think that might be one of the reasons why the patient is sick.

The patient was even more disgusting than the house. He was covered in his own excrement. His skin was dotted with AIDS related skin cancer. His arm had a large cut on it that had closed, but not before it became infected. It looked like gangrene was setting in. And to top things off, maggots were crawling around under his skin.

"What's the problem?" The crew asked the patient's

friend, who was not much better at hygiene.

"You've got to get him out of here."

"Why?"

"What do you mean *why*? Look at him! He's disgusting!" *He's disgusting? People in a shit ridden, rodent infested glass house shouldn't throw stones!*

Did I hear you right? Did you say you want another death and decaying story? Ok!

A Jersey City man was watching TV in his living room when he felt something wet drip on his head. He looked up and saw a little wet spot on the ceiling tiles. Not thinking anything of it since the apartment above usually leaks when the man takes a shower, he went on watching the baseball game. Forgetting about the dripping, he sprawled out on the couch and went to sleep.

He woke up a few hours later and he was wet. The dripping had gotten worse. His upper body was soaked. The liquid smelled nasty, so he thought the toilet had overflowed. He went up to the apartment above to confront the man. He knocked on the door, but no one answered. He checked around and found that the man's car was still outside. Getting worried, he called for an ambulance.

The Fire Department first responders arrived within minutes. They received the go-ahead from the building owner and the police to force entry into the apartment. They broke through the first door and the smell was overwhelming. They traced the smell back to the bathroom and tried to open the door. It was unlocked, but wouldn't budge more than an inch or two. They could see the man's foot through the gap and decided some alterations were needed.

They cut a hole in the wall next to the door and made their way in. The resident of the apartment was sitting on the toilet, slumped over so that his head was resting on the back of the door. That was what prevented them from entering the bathroom. It appeared that the man had been dead for a few days. Neither the toilet nor the bathtub had overflowed. The liquid dripping on the man below was the combination of bodily fluids that were draining from the man's body and seeping through the floor.

My partner and I were eating lunch when a man who looked like he was in pain approached us. I knew by the way he was shuffling that we were in for a real nasty treat. "You guys gotta help me!" He was almost in tears as he spoke.

"Well, what's wrong?" In retrospect, I know I would have been a lot happier had I not asked that question, but there was no way around it.

"I have these things on my ass."

"What kind of 'things?'"

"I don't know, but they're burning and bleeding."

"Hemorrhoids?"

"No, they're something else." *Well, if you don't know what they are, how can you say for certain that they're not hemorrhoids?* "You wanna take a look?"

"No, that's okay, sir."

"No, no. Take a look."

"Sir, I will take your word for it. What hospital can I take you to?"

"No! Here!" He yelled, attracting a crowd. "Look at it!"

"Sir, that's okay..."

"No, look!" At that, he dropped his pants and practically shoved his ass in my face. *And I thought his top half smelled nasty.* I tried to avert my eyes, but it was too late. The image of a hairy, dirty ass will be forever burned into my memory.

My worst nightmare almost came true. I hate riding in elevators. I'm not necessarily afraid of small places, but I hate elevators. To make matters worse, I often have to ride in the elevators in housing projects. Anyone who has worked in housing projects knows what I am talking about - they're all the same.

There are two stairways: one is kept clean and the other is used as a bathroom. The clean one, not to sound stereotypical, is where drug dealers usually set up shop. The elevators are *always* covered in urine when you step into them. Why? I haven't got a clue. I have a Bachelor's Degree in sociology and still I can't figure this one out.

I was dispatched to a housing project for a sick child. The apartment was on the 12th floor, *and I'll be damned if I was going to walk up 12 flights of stairs,* so we took the elevator. On the way down, my worse fear almost came true – the elevator stopped. I swore that if I ever got stuck in one of the project elevators I would kill myself rather than suffocate to the smell of stale urine.

I tried to remain calm because I like life and didn't feel like checking out yet. I called on my radio for help but the radio wouldn't transmit in the elevator shaft. Now was the time to panic. I pounded on the walls and yelled at the top of my lungs. Yelling only made things worse because I had to inhale the ammonia-like stench in order to yell some more. Finally, in desperation, I made my peace with God, rolled up my sleeves and got ready to gnaw through my wrists like a trapped animal. Luckily for me, the elevator began to move again just as I was about to clamp down on my radial arterial.

I responded to a welfare motel in Lawrenceville for a sick person. (*Is it me or does there seem to be a lot of sick people in this chapter?*) When I arrived I found a lady lying in the fetal position on the edge of her bed. She was throwing up large chunks of something green. *Don't know what, don't want to know what.*

Some police officers responded to help us, so there were

eight people crammed into this little room. We were interviewing the patient with the door open, *to let the smell out*, when a man came up to the door. He looked in for a moment, then walked away. We didn't think any of it, figuring he was just a curious onlooker.

We were going about our business when he came back a minute or two later. The lady was still on the bed throwing up, the place smelled horrible, and there were four police officers and three EMTs in the room. Despite all of those things the man walked right between everyone and lay down next to the lady on the bed.

"Sir," a police officer asked, "is this your room?"

"Nope." With that he rolled over on the bed and went to sleep.

I responded for an unknown medical emergency. When I arrived and walked up the stairs, I found the patient lying in the fetal position on the bed. He was having uncontrollable diarrhea. It looked like someone left the tap on at the ice cream store. It was all swirling into a pile on the floor by the bed.

The worst part was the flies – a cloud of them like a scene from *The Amityville Horror*. I was trying my best to keep from throwing up. However, as I approached the patient, one of the flies buzzed into my ear. I immediately lost it and commenced to do the 'Fly-in-the-Ear Dance.' For those that have never seen it (which is probably everyone reading this except my partner), run around in circles, flailing your arms and swinging at your ear, screaming "It's in my ear! It's in my ear. Sweet Jesus, it's in my ear!"

I got it out and spent a few minutes composing myself as my partner assessed the patient. From the spaced out look on the patient's face, we figured he wouldn't be able to understand us, but it was worth a shot. "Sir, what is the problem?"

Just then, his wife yelled in from the other room. "Ah, baby, he can't hear what you're saying!"

"Okay, ma'am, thank you." My partner went on assessing the patient. "Sir, we're going to take you to the hospital, okay?"

At that, the wife entered the room. "Ah, baby! He can't hardly walk!"

I turned around to tell her that we knew and we just trying to tell him what was going on. As I opened my mouth to say something, I saw that she eating a bowl full of brown slop that looked like the diarrhea. At that, I ran gasping out of the room.

This is the all-time worst thing I have ever seen. Well, it is for now. I'm sure something more nauseating is waiting around the corner for me.

I was dispatched to check on the welfare of a man. His family had not heard from him all day. His daughter called the ambulance because she had not been able to reach him by phone. Unfortunately, this usually means that the person has passed away.

On this occasion, my supervisor decided on a whim to respond with us. He arrived before and was met in the lobby of the building by the man's daughter. She didn't have any keys, and a superintendent could not be found, so the police Emergency Services' Unit was called. I arrived and we all made our way upstairs.

The chief knocked on the door and yelled inside. At first there was no response. Then, very faintly, we could hear someone moaning for help. He said that he couldn't get up. As soon as the ESU arrived they knocked down the door with a battering ram. And what a sight was there for us on the other side of the door.

Mind you, the daughter said that she hadn't been able to get a hold of him *that* day. She said she talked to him yesterday. I really don't think so. Someone was fibbing to me.

The patient was lying face down on the hardwood floor of his dining room. Shockingly, he was still breathing and moaning weakly. A horrendous odor filled the air. It was a mix of feces, urine, bile, sweat, and vomit. He was lying in a puddle of his own wastes. I threw two pairs of gloves on and attempted to roll him over. I couldn't move him and he let out a terrible cry.

Upon closer examination, we found that the waste products had solidified and glued him to the floor. There were also clumps of hardened feces around the floor, as well as one that was stuck trying to exit his body. There was absolutely no way his daughter could have talked to him yesterday. He had to have been on that floor for a couple of days.

Thinking quickly, my chief told us to mix some soap and water and pour it on the floor. After doing that, we had to slowly move him back and forth to try to break the cell. Once he was loose, we were able to roll him on to his back. Large pieces of skin ripped off as we rolled him over. Other areas of skin had begun to break down from the pressure of being in that position for an extended period of time. Every time we tried to take his blood pressure or move him, more pieces of skin would slough off.

Now that I have written that, I am really not looking forward to what work holds for me.

HARMON AND CRESCENT

21:03 Hours

"What do you think the odds are that this guy got up and left?" My partner says apathetically as he looks out the passenger side window at the sidewalk.

"We should be so lucky." Without thinking, I turn down the radio so I can concentrate on looking for my patient. I smile when I realize how ridiculous that is.

We were dispatched to the intersection of Harmon Street and Crescent Avenue for a report of a "man down." That category of patients usually turns out to be drunks, who we can wake up, or dead bodies. We're hoping for either – *less carrying and paperwork involved*!

I slow down as we approach the area. I turn off the lights so we don't attract too much attention. Large crowds are never good. We look around and see nothing. I'm all set to call back in service when someone runs into the middle of the street waving at us.

I roll down my window only far enough to hear, but not let out the cold air from my AC. "Mistah," the young lady says, "He over there." She points to an area a little further up the street, closer to the intersection of Harmon and Monticello.

"Thanks," I sigh as I park the truck in the middle of the street. I turn on the rear light bar in a vain attempt to ward off drivers from coming down this street. It doesn't do the trick. They see the flashing lights and still turn down the one-way street. Once they get to the back of my truck, they start honking for me to move. It doesn't bother me much anymore; I actually take comfort in the fact that I am inconveniencing them.

Someone yells at my partner to move. He responds by waving at the driver with exaggerated kindness. We walk towards our patient. A body lies slumped between a large oak tree and a chain link fence. The patient looks like a young black man in his mid twenties and very muscular. He's lying with his back to us, but his white tank top shows off his bulging physique. Black ink tattoos adorn his shoulders.

From where I am standing, I can see that he's still breathing. Instinctively, my partner and I put on our leather work gloves at the same time. I extend my foot and tap him a gently in the small of his back. He stirs, but then doesn't move. I assume a safety position — lowering my head to protect my windpipe and kneeling so that my left leg is in front of my privates — and grab his shoulder and roll him onto his back. He moves without protest and lies still with his eyes closed. A thick glob of saliva is clinging to the corner of his mouth. I make a fist and start rubbing forcefully on his sternum to wake him up. It has the desired effect.

His eyes snap open and he yells. In an instant he is on his feet and backing himself against the fence. He moves so fast that it takes me by surprise. However, in that instant I catch a whiff of something bad. It is a medicinal smell and it instantly takes me back to my freshman year of college and dissecting a cat in Anatomy class. He's been smoking formaldehyde – "Dip," as it's called on the street – and it makes him very unstable. Definitely not a person I want to mess with.

"Why do all the Dip heads have to be weightlifters, too?" I look over my shoulder and see that the police Emergency Services has arrived. I breathe a sigh of relief. These guys are like the old west cavalry, specially trained, and if needed, they have pepper spray and stun guns.

The patient looks around, wildly turning his head back and forth. His eyes don't move, but look straight ahead wherever his head moves. More drool escapes his mouth and he breathes with increasingly deep breaths. As the police move closer, his respirations increase. Sweat beads shine on his head, illuminated by the streetlight above us. The number of beads increases as his breathing gets faster. He moves his head more rapidly, plotting an escape.

He yells and charges directly at me. Maybe he thinks I'm the least muscular of the group, or maybe he senses that I don't care about him and could care less if he gets run over by a car and therefore am the mostly likely to get out of his way and let him run. Whatever his reasoning, if there is any, I find myself watching this beast of a man run at me in a surreal slow motion. In that slow motion, I pray for police intervention. And in that same slow motion, I watch as his baggy black jean shorts fall from around his waist and trip him up. He falls flat on his face and we all pile on top of him.

The police cuff him and put shackles on him to double the restraint. We lead him to the back of the ambulance where he commences to cry and sob the entire way to the hospital. I can't help but wonder that this is the same man who would have snapped me in two just moments earlier.

PSYCHIATRIC EMERGENCIES

I was called to assist the local police with a transport to a crisis center. There were a couple of police officers standing around inside of this house, all with their hands in their pockets. That caused me to let my guard down a little.

There was a female in her twenties sitting on the couch. She looked very agitated. Her mother stood in the corner crying.

"What's the problem?" I asked one of the police officers. He just shrugged and gestured towards the young lady. "Okay." I turned my attention to her. "Ma'am, what's wrong?"

She suddenly jumped out of the chair and dove for me. Before I knew what was going on, she had latched herself onto my arm and wouldn't let go. "Don't make me go back there! Don't make me go back!"

"Please let go of me." I tried to pry her off, and the officers were still standing in the corner. "Go back where?"

"Back to that school!" She then told me she was a teacher in a Trenton school and that the kids had "driven her crazy."

Then she started to laugh. "You see this, is all part of my plan."

"Your plan?"

"Yeah. See I'm working on a thesis paper on how people react to crazy people and you are all part of this." From the look of shock on the mother's face, I would venture to say that the patient wasn't being very truthful with me. "Okay, now that you have all helped me, you can be on your way." She started ushering me towards the door.

"All right!" An officer finally stepped in. "Cut the crap. We know you're lying. Let's go to the hospital." He took her by the arm and started to drag her to the ambulance.

"No! I will not go back!" She started flailing her arms and crying. Inside the ambulance, she grabbed my partner's thigh in a death grip. "Don't let them take me back. This is all part of a test!"

"Ma'am, please let go of my partner," I asked nicely and she did. "Please keep your hands off of us."

"Okay." She seemed sincere. That is, until she hauled off and slapped my partner. "Don't get mad at me, this is all for a paper!"

I gotta hand it to her. If she was crazy, she made up a good story. And if she was telling us the truth, it *was* one hell of an experiment.

I responded for a nonviolent EDP. A man was standing near a payphone smoking a cigarette. He snubbed it out and walked up to us when we stepped out of the truck. He introduced himself and said that he was depressed and wanted to kill himself. He decided on which hospital he wanted us to take him to and we opened the back door for him.

Just before he stepped into the ambulance, "Abraca-dabra!" He called out and launched into this weird ritual dance. He snapped his fingers twice, then clapped his hands twice, and finally patted himself frantically all over. "I'm invisible!" He called out with glee.

I looked at my partner with disbelief, and we stood there for a moment not saying anything. "Holy shit!" My partner called out. "Where'd he go?"

The patient started laughing, then did the ritual again. "Abracadabra! I'm back!"

"My god!" I said in a sarcastic voice. "That's something. How did you do that?"

"You wanna see it again?" Once more he did the ritual.

"Wow, I can't see you." My partner said with a straight face. "Can you make yourself visible again so we can get going?"

The man walked in the ambulance and did the ritual dance. He was laughing loudly, "Bet you didn't see me walk by, did ya?"

"No," I said. "You gotta stop that. I need to be able to see you."

We drove to the hospital and walked him inside. The ER was crowded and it suddenly dawned on him that he would have to wait for a while. He didn't like that too much. "Time to split!" He did the dance and tried to run for the door. My partner reached out, grabbed him by the back of the neck and pinned him against the wall. "How did you get me?"

"Lucky guess."

I responded for a 'man down' in Jersey City. That usually means that an intoxicated person has fallen asleep in public or the person calling doesn't feel like checking to see if the body is unconscious. When we arrived, a police officer met us with a smile. "I know *you're* gonna love this," she said as she gave me a playful punch in the arm.

"I know I probably won't, but go ahead."

"She's a bit of a nut to begin with, but she's been doing

heroin today."

"Nice."

"Well, that ain't the best part."

Just as she said that, her partner walked the patient past me into the ambulance. I caught a whiff of feces and almost threw up. "Did she shit herself?"

"Kinda." The officer was cracking herself up.

"What?"

"She was taking a shit, but then she put it in her pockets."

"Are you serious?"

"Do you want to check?"

I looked at the patient and saw brown stains on her white pants. That was all I needed to see. I hung my head and moaned. I had to be in the back with her.

On the way to the hospital, she kept nodding off because of the heroin. When I yelled at her, she woke up. We reached the hospital and she nodded off in the parking lot. "Ma'am get up! Let's go! Come on!" My partner was yelling at her and grabbed her arm.

She woke up and looked around lethargically. "You don't have to get nasty!"

"Nasty?" I said, "Ma'am, you're well beyond that."

The dispatcher radioed me, "You're responding to Monticello and Harrison for the female running around in traffic."

"Three-fifteen received. Do you have a description?"

"Sure. She *should* be the only one running around naked, six months pregnant."

"Ugh, received. At least she won't be hard to spot."

As we rounded the corner onto Harrison Ave, we were met by a police car. "Where's the patient?" I asked. They simply pointed to a woman walking across the street in the rain. She was wearing a soaked dress. "She put on clothes?"

"Yeah, she was bare-ass naked before," one of the officers said, "but we made her put some clothes on."

"God bless you two."

As we approached her, she started to run. We caught up to her and the police forced her into the back of the ambulance. She began screaming, "You can't make me go back to the hospital!"

"What were you in the hospital for?" I asked.

"Hospital?" She sounded confused. "I wasn't in the hospital. Who told you I was in the hospital?"

"You did."

"When?"

"Just now."

"No I didn't!"

"Yes, you did."

Thankfully, before this became an all night thing, my partner jumped in. "Doesn't matter, let's go to the hospital."

On the way I began to interview her. She wouldn't provide me with any information, and I was getting a little annoyed. "Are you suicidal?"

"No."

"Are you depressed? Do you need a hug?"

"No."

In my best Elvis Presley, "Are you lonesome tonight?"

After that, she just began to ramble on when I asked her questions. I would never get any answer, just a long, meaningless dissertation. Finally, I gave up, but there were a few things I wanted to know.

"What are your feelings on the gas crisis? Is peace in the Middle East possible? Do you support the adoption of children by homosexual couples? How many oranges are in a week?"

I had just gotten into work when my stomach started rumbling. Realizing that it always wise to obey the master, my partner and I decided on where we would eat lunch and headed for a deli near a busy subway station.

As we pulled up, we saw another ambulance parked across the street. I waved, although I was pretty sure they didn't see me. We walked in and tried to get something to eat. Just as I went to order, I heard one of the people on the crew across the street scream into the radio. "Dispatcher, call the police, they have an officer in need of assistance!"

My girlfriend had just dumped me and the coordinator had just yelled at my partner for something, so we were in the fighting mood. I looked at him, he looked at me, and we both shrugged. Positive we were thinking the same thing, I asked, "Bar fight?"

"Bar fight," he answered.

We jumped in the ambulance and tore across four lanes of traffic. We saw an officer struggling to subdue a man, trying to fend him off with one hand and call for back up with the other. We surprised the hell out of both men when we drove up on the curb and nearly ran them both over.

Before I had the ambulance in park, my partner was out and jumping on the guy's back. I ran over and grabbed his legs. Together we hoisted him up in the air and pinned him face down on the sidewalk. I threw myself on his back until the officer handcuffed him.

I looked up in time to see my tour chief barreling down the road towards us. He had heard the other crew screaming and thought they were in trouble. He didn't look like he was about to stop, and I felt what the cop must have felt: I nearly crapped my pants.

Just then, the bystander I had been waiting for piped in. You know the one I'm talking about: the conspiracy theorist who didn't see a thing, but already knew why it happened. "You can't treat that man like that! You're only doing that cause you're white and he's black." With that, several other bystanders who must have been watching another fight chimed in with slurs that we were all racists.

Finally, after enduring as much mindless insults as he could take, my partner looked dramatically at his hands for a moment, then stood up on a bench and yelled, "Last time I looked I was black!" That dispersed the crowd very nicely.

As it turned out though, the man we helped subdue had an extensive, violent psychiatric history and several warrants against him for stalking and assaulting the two female EMTs on the crew that initially called for assistance. He also had a warrant for assaulting the ambulance itself.

I was sent to a private house for a violent EDP. When we arrived, the police were leading a lady out of the house in handcuffs. Another officer followed close behind with a sledgehammer in his hands.

The officer with the tool had a wide grin on his face. "Oh, you'll love this!" *That's always a great way to start things off.* "She just walked into this house and started swinging the sledgehammer."

"At who?"

"At the walls. Doing renovations."

"You've got to be kidding me?"

"Nope. She said she wants to make a school."

"Really?" I asked. "Public or private?"

"Does it matter?" The officer said with a laugh.

"Only for state funding, I guess," I quipped back.

Can you just imagine being the homeowners? You're sitting in your living room watching TV and a lady you've never seen before comes in and starts destroying your house with a sledgehammer. *I would have paid to see that!*

I was dispatched to the parking lot of a shopping mall to assist the police. As I arrived, I saw more police officers than I thought the department had surrounding a man who was kneeling on a grassy island by the main road. He had prostrated himself and was praying. *Oh yeah, and he was naked in December.*

The police had succeeded in getting the man to allow them to handcuff him and, *mercifully for me,* wrap a sheet around him. We walked him to the ambulance and the police asked me if there was a more comfortable way of restraining him. I said sure and began securing him with triangular bandages. That's when he wigged out.

He started screaming and trying to swing at me. "I am the king! You are all shit!" He continued yelling in my good ear that he was the king until I couldn't take it anymore.

"Sir, might I remind you that there was only one king and he died for your sins in 1977." That statement shut *everyone* up in the back of the ambulance. Suddenly, everyone was looking at me with confused looks on their faces. "What? No one ever heard of Elvis?" For the remainder of the call we called him Mr. Presley because he didn't want to tell us his real name. *What can I say? I have a soft spot for Elvis.*

When he became violent as we tried to get him into the ambulance, we had to restrain him. As I was tying him down with the aid of some police officers, he began growling at me and trying to bite me. "Elvis, knock it off," I keep demanding politely. Thinking there was a chance he was on some type of drug, I tried to check his pupils. When I looked closer, he lunged forwards and tried to bite me again. "Try that again and I'm going to treat you like a dog." I went to look again and he tried to bite me again. "Look, I know you can understand me. Do that again and I'll pop you in the nose!" Once more I tried, and once more he growled and tried to bite me. So I rolled up a stack of run reports and smacked him in the nose like I would my dog.

I arrived at an apartment for a possible stroke and was met at the door by the patient. After interviewing her, we came to the conclusion that she was probably not having a stroke. She called because she had a cramp in her foot and our idiot dispatcher decided that meant she was having a stroke. *I guess she said she was* really *having a cramp in her foot.*

Finding that was the problem, I probably should have left it at that till I got outside, but while she was getting her shoes together I asked her if anything else was bothering her. "Oh yeah," she said matter-of-factly, "my breasts are milking."

"I'm sorry, what?"

"I'm lactating from my breasts." *Lactating from my breasts seems a bit redundant 'cause I would hate to think of where else you could lactate.*

For some reason, that struck me as a funny statement. To make matters worse, upon hearing this, my partner started making milking gestures on his chest behind the patient's back. Trying my best to maintain composure, I stepped outside the apartment for some fresh air. I looked up at the door directly across the hall and completely lost it. I doubled over and started laughing hysterically to the point I was crying.

Taped to the door across the hall was a "Got Milk?" ad.

I don't know if this guy was really crazy, but I hope, for his sake, he was. If not, he's just an asshole.

I was dispatched to the Port Authority Police Desk at Journal Square to decontaminate a patient who was sprayed with OC Spray. When we arrived, I could hear him yelling from down the hall. "I am outraged at this! I am outraged! You can't treat me like this!"

I met one of the PATH ESU officers in the hall who told me the man had been arrested for shouting on a PATH train that he wanted to shoot everyone. *I don't know why, but to me that sounded like a pretty reasonable excuse to arrest someone.*

As we were getting the whole story, I could still hear him in the other room. "You can't strip search me! I know my rights! It's in the Constitution!"

"Sir," one of the officers asked, "where in the Constitution is it written?"

"I don't know, but I know it's in there. You can't strip search me!"

"Sir, I am just removing your jacket and patting you down. I am not strip searching you, but I am within the law should I decide to strip search you."

This went on for a few minutes. After a while I couldn't understand what was being said with all the shouting. Then I heard all I needed to hear to know this wasn't going to be pretty. One of the officers yelled at him, "Oh, you think you can push me in my house?" Before I knew what was going on, my eyes were burning and everyone around me was coughing. One of the officers emerged from the room with a canister of OC spray the size of a fire extinguisher.

His eyes burning, the man was screaming. I waited a few more minutes until the irritating mist dispersed and it was okay to open my eyes; then I went inside to talk to the patient.

"What's the problem?"

"You're only doing this because I am black!"

"Sir, I haven't done anything to you yet. But I can assure you that's only because you haven't been calm enough to let me near you."

"I am outraged!"

"Sir, what is you're name?"

"I am outraged!"

"Okay, Mr. Raged, do you have any medical problems?"

"I am an asthmatic," and as an afterthought, "I'm having trouble breathing."

I had my partner check his lungs because I was concerned he would have an attack. My partner said his lungs were clear. "Sir, I am going to flush your eyes out now."

"I don't trust you."

"Why? What have I done to you?"

"Because you're white."

"Sir, I am just going to put some water in your eyes."

"I am outraged!" *Oh no, not this again.* "You can't lock me up like this!"

"Sir, please stop yelling. You threatened to shoot everyone on a PATH train; you're lucky they only maced you. Do you have any medical problems? High blood pressure, diabetes, psychiatric problems?"

"No."

"Have you taken any drugs tonight?"

"Why are you asking that? Is it because I'm a black man? Do you think that all black men take drugs?"

"No, because I think you're an asshole and I hope that you don't normally act like this." That shut him up.

We checked his blood pressure and got some more information. Then he began complaining of having trouble breathing again. Once again, I had my partner listen to his lungs. "They sound fine to me," he said, offering me his stethoscope. "But if you want to listen, go right ahead. Maybe I missed something."

"That's okay. I'm deaf anyway. If you didn't hear, I sure as hell won't."

"How can they hire you if you're deaf?" The patient asked me.

Almost at my wits' end, I said sarcastically, "Because I wasn't deaf when I was hired, a tumor destroyed my hearing (*which is the God's honest truth*), so if they try to fire me I'll have a nice discrimination lawsuit." He looked at me with disbelief. "It's in the Constitution. Right next to where it says you can't be strip searched for threatening to shoot up a crowded train."

At that he spat on me, to which the ESU responded by spraying him a third time. "Now, Stupid, are you going to let me treat you or do you want to be maced a fourth time?"

He began shaking his hands in a gesture for me to help him. "Okay sir, tilt your head back."

"Wait, how do I know what you're putting in my eyes?"

"Because I told you it's just water."

"How do I know that?"

"Because it says right here on the bottle. See? Distilled Sterile Water."

"I can't read that! They maced me, remember?"

"Then just let me wash your eyes out and you can read for yourself."

Finally, we convinced him to allow us to rinse his eyes out. "Do you want us to take you to the hospital?"

"No."

I handed him the clipboard with the refusal sheet. "Sir, please sign where the X is."

"What's that supposed to mean? You think you a black man can't sign his full name, that he has to sign an X instead?"

"Look, you lousy, racist bastard!" I was trying to suppress my desire to belt him. "Just sign your name where I marked an X and let me get the hell away from you!"

"You don't have to be so rude about it."

It's a wonder I haven't completely lost my mind on a call yet!

A police officer friend once told me how to deal with people like this. After they've been sprayed and are screaming at you and being an all-around obnoxious pain in the butt, spray more OC spray onto a rag and hand it to them. Tell them it's the antidote and watch the fun begin.

I was dispatched to pick up one of my regulars one evening. "Tony" is one of my favorites. He's not a nasty drunk, and usually doesn't smell *that* bad. He goes through these phases in the way he dresses. He'll wear a blue leisure suit for a while – his Elvis phase. Then he'll wear jeans, a vest, and a bandanna – his Willie Nelson look.

I went to pick him up, and much to my surprise and later chagrin, he brought along a friend—"Al." Since Tony is one of our regulars, I had photocopied his chart so I don't have to bother with extracting information from him when he is one of his incredibly drunken states. As, I had never met Al before, I had to interview him.

"What's your name?"

"My name is Al."

"Okay, Al. How are you?"

He looked at me with a dumbfounded expression. "My name is Al."

"I know. Al, we covered that. How old are you?"

"I'm Al."

"Okay." I could feel something pulsating behind my eye, so I figured I should try another approach before I had a stroke. "When is your birthday?"

"I'm thirty-six."

That pulsating sensation just turned into a pounding crescendo. "Do you have any medical problems?"

"I was born August eighth."

I looked at my partner, whose mouth was wide open with amazement, and just cracked up. "How many questions do I have to lead him with in order to get the answer I'm looking for?"

I was dispatched for a person with difficulty walking at a Port Authority Subway station. When I arrived, I saw a lady sitting in a wheelchair, with a half a dozen bags, waving for us. I asked her what the problem was in my usual jovial manner.

"I was on the PATH train heading for Newark and I had to get off in Jersey City because I couldn't go any further."

"What do you mean you couldn't go any further?"

"My legs felt weak, like they were going to go out on me."

I looked at my partner, and she looked at me, and silently we came to the same conclusion: someone had to say it. So say it we did at the same time. "Ma'am, you realize you're in a wheelchair, right?"

"Yes. I realize that."

Almost at the same time again, we asked, "And you do realize that wheelchair is on a *moving* train, right?"

"But I just couldn't go on any further."

Okay, terrific! Moving right along...

I asked her for identification and she gave me a hospital card from a hospital in New York City. "Is this still your home address on the card?"

"Yes, it is."

"What hospital do you want to go to tonight?"

"Can you take me to (a city hospital) because I heard that they shelter the homeless."

"But ma'am," my partner interjected, "you're homeless, but you still have an address in New York City?"

"Yes, that's where I get my mail."

What I want to know is who's living there now and what do they think when she shows up to collect her mail? More importantly, what sort of mail does she get? If it's Victoria's Secret catalogs...

So we finished doing what we had to do and began to move her to the ambulance. Dinner was getting cold, so of course we wanted to expedite her transport to the hospital. My partner started to push her out to the ambulance in the wheelchair.

"Wait!" The urgency in her voice stopped us dead in our tracks.

"What's the problem ma'am?"

"You're pushing too fast. I'm getting short of breath."

"What?"

"I can't breathe when you push so fast."

"Wait," I don't think I've ever been more confused, "you get short of breath when *we* push *you* in a *wheelchair*?"

"Yes."

"Ma'am, it's physiologically impossible for *you* to get worn out when *I'm* doing all of the work."

"Boy," my partner said nonchalantly to me, "if I had a dime for every time I've said that..."

Paranoid schizophrenics are usually the most fun, especially when they present with conspiracy theories. I've tried my hand at writing fiction and I have never been able to come up with plots as unique as some of these.

I had a patient tell me that the big oil companies of the world were working together to run a prostitution ring in Las Vegas. But they were also getting help from Sprint Long Distance and the Bell Atlantic Yellow Pages. Her sixteen-year-old daughter was the main hooker in the prostitution ring, so that was why she smuggled her illegally across state lines. I would have *totally* dismissed this as ludicrous had the police not also arrested her daughter and found a dozen hotel keys from Las Vegas in her purse. *See, it all makes perfect sense if you think about it.*

I learned an important lesson about conspiracy theories in the wake of the World Trade Center disaster: there may actually be some truth to what these people are saying.

A few months before 9-11, I sat with a suicidal patient hanging from a fire escape on the sixth floor of her building for almost twelve hours. She was screaming that the federal government had tapped her phones, someone was watching her, and her boyfriend was trying to kill her. She kept demanding a cell phone so that we could let her speak to her boyfriend.

Of course, we didn't. Rule number one of dealing with suicidal patients: never give them a cell phone or bring in the person they are demanding. Usually they are calling for these people so that this person can witness the suicide. Instead, the police set up airbags to catch her if she jumped. Then we waited. There was a $100 pool going among some of the cops to see if she would jump/fall, be talked in, or be forcibly dragged in. I bet she'd be talked in.

I lost. (As if I could ever win anything.) After eleven hours, fifty-three minutes, and forty-two seconds (but hey, who's counting), she was yanked from her precarious position by a brave police officer.

Either she was completely insane or she was one of the more sane people I have ever encountered: a day or two after the World Trade Center was attacked, her boyfriend was arrested in connection with the terrorism investigation.

Bored out of my mind one evening, I decided to meet my friend at the ER and give him a hand with his violent EDP. He is generally calm on the radio, so I figured it had to be good when I could hear excitement in his voice. Just for effect, his partner keyed up the radio just as the lady was screaming "Fuck you, motherfuckers! I'll kill all of you!"

They pulled up and I opened the back to remove the stretcher. She started cursing me, saying that I had beaten her up. I had never seen her before. She was handcuffed to the stretcher, but was still kicking and screaming. We wheeled her down the hall, past hordes of amused onlookers.

She was cursing loudly, so my friend attempted to calm her down. "I thought you and me were cool. C'mon. Calm down a little."

She looked at my friend and smiled. "Oh, yeah, we cool. You my head dog."

I swear I thought she said something different. So turned to my friend and said, "What? You gave her head?" With that, she flipped out and started cursing and calling me stupid.

"What school did you go to?" She asked.

"I'm working on a master's, thank you very much," I answered smugly.

"Well I got a master's too, but it ain't legal!" *I was* not *expecting* that*!* I have to give it to her. That really ended the argument fast. I couldn't think of anything to come back with.

"You think that's confusing," a cop said to me as he looked over my shoulder. "She swears she's my mother."

Another crew was dispatched to a senior citizen's high-rise for a non violent EDP. When they arrived, the patient was cowering behind his bed. "Sir, what's the problem?"

"Get away from the windows!" His yell took everyone by surprise and everybody ducked away from the windows.

"What?"

"Snipers!"

"I'm sorry, come again?" They asked as they pulled themselves off the floor.

"Snipers in the windows up there. They're shooting at me."

"Did they get you?" *Please, don't look at this book like that. You know you would have asked the same thing.*

"No, I managed to dodge them."

"Do you want to go to the hospital?"

"Yeah, but they'll get me if I try to walk outside."

"We'll protect you," one of the police officers said.

"Can I wear one of your vests?"

"Not a chance. But we'll help you."

Their idea of helping was to stand outside, hold the door and yell at the patient run. "Quick, zig-zag pattern. Zig-zag!" The patient followed their orders and zig-zagged his way to the back of the truck.

Luckily no one was injured by sniper fire.

One of the things they teach about dealing with psychiatric emergencies is to never play into the delusions or hallucinations. However, sometimes it's just easy than trying to reason with them.

I was greeted by a police officer as I stepped out of my ambulance. "Okay, are you guys ready for this?" *That's usually never a good sign.* "This lady thinks her husband is trying to kill her and she's refusing to leave the house. I don't know how we're going to get her out."

I walked inside and saw the lady pacing around in the kitchen. She was visibly upset and yelling. "Where's her husband?"

"He's asleep in the bedroom."

"Ma'am, what's wrong?"

"My husband's trying to kill me!"

Acting surprised, I screamed, "Oh my god! He's trying to kill you? Then let's get you somewhere safe! Hurry!" I got behind her and we ran out of the house and right into the ambulance.

The police officers looked very shocked and bewildered. "That was incredible! We've been here for a half an hour trying to get her out."

"Hey," I said nonchalantly, "I may look like I'm twelve, but I've been at this for a while."

While beginning the second half of a 24-hour shift, I was dispatched to a luxury high rise for a violent EDP. We were advised not to enter the scene without police. We responded quickly, beating the police, so I took a short nap while waiting. I awoke a half an hour later and still no sign of police. We had our dispatcher call the police back for an ETA, but we never got one.

"Bro," my partner asked, "How bad can it be?"

"I don't know. Wanna see?"

With that, we went to the twenty-fourth floor of this apartment building; effectively limiting our escape should the need arise. We listened closely before knocking. When we heard no sound, we knocked. A lady opened the door and thanked us for coming. She gestured to a young man seated on the coach.

He stood up and I pulled a muscle in my neck trying to see the top of him. He was well over seven feet tall, and about four hundred pounds. He clearly outweighed my partner and I put together. It was pretty obvious that if he went crazy, we were screwed.

I asked him what the problem was and he began explaining to me how the world was against him. "They fear me because I'm a genius. I got a fourth grade education, but I'm a genius" *Hey, who am I to argue with him?* "And I got titties but I ain't a bitch." *Once again, he's making perfect sense to me.* "I just got out of Riker's Island (a New York City prison)." *This means two things. (1) He's not our typical, everyday EDP. (2) He can pretty much say or do anything he wants to me and I'll feel no shame in not putting up a fight... so long as I make it home alive at the end of the day. I'm not a proud man.*

Somehow we managed to talk him into going peacefully to the hospital. En route though, my partner somehow got lost and it began pissing off our patient. Thankfully, he tried to stand up and knocked his head against the ceiling, stunning him long enough to calm him down.

Sometimes it pays to wait for the police.

I love working with new partners just to see the look on their faces when they encounter real EDPs for the first time. I was working with a new guy who couldn't have been more than nineteen years old – *listen to me trying to sound like an old fart* – and we were dispatched to pick up one of our frequent visitors.

We arrived to find multiple police officers crowded in her small apartment. "Where is she?" I asked.

"She's in the shower," an officer informed me.

"The shower?"

"Yeah, it makes her harder to grab when she's wet."

"I never thought I would do this, but can we please ask her *not* to shower."

Finally the police were able to get her out. She stormed past everyone and charged right out to the ambulance muttering to herself. Usually, I find it's best to just let them mutter and not engage in conversation. However, some things one must learn on one's own.

"What was that?" My partner asked.

"I said," she was very loud at this point, "Fuck them motherfuckers who think they can get a piece of me. Everyone gets a piece of me but only if I let them. And everyone's eaten my period, and still come back for more and do you know why? Because my shit is good."

I could see in the rearview mirror that his face was almost identical to what I imagine your face to be right now. "Oh, my god," he gasped to himself.

"God?" *I guess he was a little too loud.* "God's got nothing to do with this. And you know something. Jesus is not God's son. Oh, He came from God, *or so I'm told*, but He can't have none of this. Oh yeah! God can have this anytime He wants, but not Jesus. Fuck no." She stood up and started unbuckling her pants. "You want this, God?" Then turning to my partner, "Oh, you can have some too if you want!"

"No ma'am, that's okay. Please sit down." He sounded on the verge of tears.

"When God wants the booty, God just takes the booty!" *And that my friends, is the message of today's Gospel. When God wanteth the booty, God taketh the booty.*

ON PATROL IN SOUTH ZONE

22:39 Hours

The South Zone is crowded tonight as we drive around our response area. Pressure to improve response times has led our administrators to institute a policy of mobile ambulances. We have no "comfort station" to return to when we're done with a job, only our ambulance.

The area we're covering is the tough section of the city. Drugs and gangs are prevalent, keeping both EMS and police busy. So far this evening, things have been relatively quiet by usual standards. I have the window rolled down, taking in the sounds and smells of the area.

As we drive down Martin Luther King Drive, the smell of ribs and chicken barbecuing fill the ambulance. On the corner of MLK and Claremont Avenue, a man is cooking on a large kettledrum grill. A group of customers mill about, waiting for their orders to be ready. Pedestrians meander carelessly across the stretch, causing traffic to stop periodically. A little further up the road, young men in low-riders are double parked trying to impress young ladies.

Music is blaring from several different stereos, including our own.

My partner's eyes scan back and forth across the street as he smiles and talks to me. "So there we are, this guy's in the tub still actively seizing. His wife or girlfriend, or whoever she was, is standing over my shoulder screaming at us to do something. I try to calmly tell her we can't do much until he stops seizing. She again screams at me to do something.

"So Mike jumps in and tells her, 'I got an idea! Go get me some soap, we'll throw a load of clothes in the tub with him and do some laundry.'" I start laughing. It's an old joke, but I'm easily amused.

I catch a glimpse of some commotion out of the corner of my eye. I turn my head just in time to see a bright burst of light. My mind registers what it is even before I hear the sound. *Pop, pop, pop, pop.*

"Shit!" I duck down into my seat. The gunshots are so close to the ambulance that I think I can feel bursts of heat with every shot. I hear screaming coming from the crowd on the street. I venture a look and see dozens of people running towards us. All around us, car alarms are sounding in a deafening blur of noise.

"Was that what I think it was?" My partner asks. I hope it's a rhetorical question. Someone answers it anyway. *Pop, pop, pop.* My partner steps on the gas and speeds down the street.

I am amazed to see people almost outrunning the ambulance. As we pull away, I hear a loud sound similar to someone slowly ripping a pair of pants.

"Bro," my partner yells, "that sounded an awful lot like a MAC-Ten to me!"

We duck down the closest side street and collect ourselves. More shots can be heard in the distance. "Three-Zero-Nine to dispatch," I try to remain calm on the radio, but my voice is quivering. "Notify police we have multiple shots fired at Wilkinson and MLK!"

The dispatcher seems more excited than I am. "Nine, is there anyone shot?"

"I don't know. Multiple shots fired, multiple people screaming and running. We're standing by in the area. I'll get you an update when I can."

"Good idea Three-Zero-Nine. We're notifying police now."

My partner slowly drives the ambulance up Stegman towards Martin Luther King. We're still a block from MLK, but I can see people running frantically about. Their screams are audible over the car alarms.

Already on edge, a *yelp* from a siren makes me jump in my seat. A police car blows past us. He's joined by another car speeding up MLK. My partner begins to drive down Stegman when he is forced to pull out of the way by the Emergency Services Truck barreling up the street behind us.

Not wanting to run into a dangerous scene, my partner waits a few minutes to give police time to secure the area. Slowly we approach. ESU officers in full tactical gear wave us in. The presence of trained police officers with automatic weapons makes me feel slightly more comfortable.

The scene is chaotic. The police, staggeringly outnumbered, try to keep family members and bystanders from running through the area. Parked cars and the sides of buildings are riddled with bullet holes. Screams of anguish and the incessant wailing of car alarms have replaced stereos. And there, in the midst of all this, is the scene I was hoping not to see.

One man is sitting against the wall of a building. He is clutching his hand to his stomach; his white shirt is soaked with blood. On the ground a few feet from him, a young woman lies on her back, motionless on the sidewalk. Bright red blood forms a large pool around her. Across the street, slumped against a bullet-ridden car, another young man is also motionless.

I do a quick assessment. The guy who's still sitting up against the wall is still alive – *for now anyway*. He's moaning, so he's still breathing. I tell my partner to see how bad he is and then to check on the female.

I run to opposite side of the street to check on the young man. I immediately can tell there is nothing I can do for him. He takes his last agonal breath as I approach. I feel for a pulse and find none. I contemplate CPR for a moment, but then I notice the blood smeared against the side of the car. Mixed in with the bloody mess are large chunks of grayish material – *brain matter*. I look at the front of his face and see one bullet hole. Considering the way people shoot around here, it's a one-in-a-million shot—right between his eyes. There's a clear entrance wound in the front, and a large gaping hole in the back of his head. *Sorry man, injuries incompatible with life...* I try not to trip over the handgun he dropped next to him.

I tell the police that the man is dead and going to be left for the medical examiner. My partner reports on his patients. He says the guy was shot twice in the abdomen. There are entrance wounds, but no exits he can see. He's losing blood, but may have a shot.

The woman is a lot worse off, he reports. She still has a pulse, but she was hit repeatedly with high velocity bullets from a MAC-10 submachine gun. Three bullets have entered her stomach, and one into her chest. Her left arm looks like it was snapped in two by one or more bullets.

I call the dispatcher and ask for more units to help. She regretfully tells me that none are available and that she'll be reaching out to another town for mutual aid. *No time to stop and be pissed off about that.*

I grab the captain of the fire engine that came to assist

and tell him I'm going to need his truck's help. Someone will have to drive our ambulance and we're going to need an extra set of hands or two in the back. His men are more than willing to help. For them, it means a commendation. For me, this job just means more paperwork and *at least* an hour of clean up.

We roll both patients onto backboards and do a half ass job securing them – I'm really not too concerned about spinal injuries when both patients are starting to circle down the drain. My patient, the female, is placed on the stretcher; my partner's, the male, is secured to the bench. Two firefighters cram into the back and assist us.

My patient is bleeding rapidly through the bandages we threw on her stomach and chest. My first course of action is to intubate my patient. It's hard to tube a patient who's secured to a backboard when you care about protecting her cervical spine. In this case, I don't care, but I still manage to only move the head slightly before the vocal cords come into view. I slide the tube in, inflate the cuff on the end of it, attach the BVM and start bagging. I see the right side of the chest rise and fall with each squeeze of the bag. A firefighter takes over ventilating while I use my stethoscope to listen to the lung sounds to make sure I placed the tube in the trachea and not the esophagus. No gurgling sounds in the belly, so I know air is going into the lungs. I cut off her top and see air bubbling in and out of the bullet wound above her left breast. I take a gauze pad and tape it down over the sucking chest wound. I leave a side loose so that air can be released as it builds up in the chest. I check the wounds to her belly and throw more dressings on.

Her blood pressure is falling fast. It's 70/40. I start an IV in her right arm – amazed at how fast I did it considering the bumpy ride the firefighter driving is putting us through. I run the fluids wide open, hoping to flood her blood stream with more fluid to replace what she lost. Sweat is streaming down my face, and stinging me as it goes into my eyes. I find another vein above where I just started the first IV, and I start another IV – running more fluid into her in a desperate effort to maintain her blood pressure. All the while, I'm well aware that this is an uphill battle I'm fighting. I look through the back windows and try to figure out where we are. I take off my gloves and call ahead to the hospital on the radio.

I'm out of breath and wiping sweat from my forehead as I call ahead. "Doc, I need the Trauma Team to the ER for two shootings." I give him a brief report and slip on another set of gloves and reassess the woman. Thankfully, her blood pressure is still maintaining where it was before.

We pull up to the ER and the back doors to the ambulance are open even before the truck is put in park. Another ambulance crew has just finished up with their patient at City General ER and stood by to help us. One EMT takes my stretcher out of the back. I climb over him to jump out and give him a hand with the stretcher. The firefighter continues to ventilate the patient as we roll the stretcher inside. The other EMT quickly slides his stretcher into our truck so they can unload the other patient.

As we pass through the doors into the Trauma Room, my heart monitor lets out a piercing beep. I know what it means before I look at the screen. She's gone into cardiac arrest. The Trauma Team moves her over to their bed and commences CPR. I give a quick report to the doctor in charge of the team, then slide out to make room for the other patient. I find a sink and spend a minute scrubbing up and washing my hands. Still wet, I run my hands through my hair and sigh.

The back of the truck is a mess. Wrappers for equipment litter the floor, red with fresh blood. Pieces of used equipment are tossed helter- skelter in around the back. The truck stinks of sweat, blood, and feces. *The contents of her bowels must have seeped out.* My partner whistles as he walks up behind me.

"Hey," he says as he pats me on the back. "They're calling your girl." As if it was something I really needed to hear, my partner continues on. "Cops say she was in the wrong place at the wrong time. She caught the spray of bullets that was intended for my guy."

I nod. I figured as much.

"We did good though." He reiterates, either to convince me or to convince himself, "Even if we couldn't save her, we *really* did. Right?"

"Yeah, I, we did," I concede. I honestly think I did the best I could have. I wipe that thought from my mind and concentrate on the important task at hand: where to start cleaning?

Expecting a funny line or a happy ending? Sorry, that's not the way it happens sometimes.

MORE STREET SLANG AND URBAN DIAGNOSES

In the following list, UD denotes *Urban Diagnosis*. SS means "Slang used by EMS providers."

AAA (SS) – *Acute Ambulance Ass.* The enlargening of your posterior due to long hours sitting on your butt or consumption of countless unhealthy meals.

ALS By Adjective and Adverb (SS) – when a call is screened as a Priority One, or life-threatening emergency, because the caller says things like "He *really* can't breath" or "This *really* hurts!"

ALS Recon (SS) – when one Advanced Life Support (ALS) paramedic gets out the truck to see if the Basic Life Support (BLS) really needs them.

Amtrax (UD) – a disease that can be used as a biological weapon, sort of like Anthrax, but in an urban environment. "*Man, he gots the Amtrax!*"

Brady-Ayes (SS) – a slow expression of discomfort, usually less than 25 'Ayes' a minute
"Aye... Aye... Aye..."

Burn Out (SS)– when someone has been at the job too long.
Levels of Burn Out:
Cajun – burnt out, but sarcastic
Crispy – completely burnt with no sense of humor

'But' Breather (SS) – a person who is unconscious, *but* breathing.

Bums Feets (UD) – when a patient's feet swell up and they can't walk.
"I gots the bums feets."

Cancelled by Intimidation (SS) – intimidating the patient to sign a refusal or a BLS unit to cancel the ALS.

Chicken Breather (SS) – a female who's in respiratory distress.
"Hey man, Che'ken breath!"

Cousins (SS) – cockroaches
"Check yourself. The cousins were all over the place."

Diabenees (UD) – Diabetes

Electric Fishes (UD)– Epileptic seizures
"He sometimes catches the electric fishes."

FTD (SS) – fixing to die

Guppy Breathing (SS) – Agonal breathing: just before a patient dies, looks like a fish gulping

HIN (SS) – Heroin Induced Narcolepsy, the intermittent nodding off to sleep as a result of taking heroin.

Incubate (UD) – when a paramedic intubates a patient with an endotracheal tube.
"One time her asthma got so bad they incubated her."

Insulation (UD) – Insulin
"I take Insulation for my Diabenees."

Kitten Stones (UD)– Kidney Stones

Lunch Box of Life (SS) – the defibrillator

Miracle Whiff (SS) – Oxygen

The Miseries (UD)– when a patient is depressed.
"I'm feeling down today. I think I got the miseries."

The Ninja (UD) – AIDS
"It's the Ninja cuz it sneaks up and kills you!"

On the Nod (SS) - the patient is on heroin, due to the classic nodding off to sleep during conversation.

PID Shuffle (SS) – the unmistakable walk associated with someone suffering from Pelvic Inflammatory Disease (PID).

Pump (UD/SS) – an inhaler for asthma or COPD.

PNT (SS) – Paramedic Nap Time.

Roaches of the Liver (UD)– Cirrhosis of the liver
"I'm dying of Roaches of the Liver."

Sickler (UD) – a person who suffers from Sickle Cell Anemia.
"She's in pain; she's a sickler!"

Status Asparagus (SS)– a persistent vegetative state

Suga–betes (UD) – Diabetes

Tachy–Ayes (SS) – a fast expression of discomfort, usually more than 25 'Ayes' a minute
"Aye, aye, aye, aye, aye, aye, aye, aye."
(Of the two, Brady-Ayes is a better indicator that something is seriously wrong.)

Tubilisscelosis (UD) - a seizure disorder. (I have no idea where they came up with this one!)

Vapors (UD) – some mysterious gas that causes ordinarily healthy people to experience anxiety attacks and pass out.
"I caught the Vapors and passed out."

MORE RANDOM THOUGHTS

"Oops" is the scariest word in healthcare.

"Healthcare Reform" is the second scariest.

Management *is* out to get you.

Stupidity is contagious.

For 80% of your calls, the only equipment you'll need is your run report and patience.

Yelling at someone *always* makes your day brighter.

Yes-ing someone to death or laughing in his face ends the fight easier that arguing with him.

A little bit of respect goes a long way, especially when you're shown none.

Your partner can be your best friend or worst enemy—twelve hours of silence is a lot longer than twelve hours of laughter.

Holding back laughter is almost as hard as holding back urination.

I'm fluent in 3 languages – English, Broken English, and Ghetto English.

It is possible to sleep in an upright position.

It is possible and sometimes necessary to completely block someone out and still appear as if you're listening. First, look at their Adam's Apple or a point on the wall just behind their head. Occasionally ask, "Oh yeah?" or repeat the last thing they said in the form of a question. Every now and then, furrow your eyebrow when you look at them, and periodically make notes (or doodlings) on your chart.

Everyone can develop a human bullshit detector.

If a situation feels wrong, it probably is.

Working hard only brings you more *work*.

No one goes to the doctor anymore, only the hospital.

If taxis entered the 911 system they would make a fortune.

Hardly anything beats the thrill of forcing someone to go to the hospital against their will, except perhaps telling someone that they'll have to wait at the hospital for a while because they are not an emergency.

Creative writing 101 is a class most EMS personnel could teach.

EMS personnel are apparently the only people who have to go to work sick or get punished for being late.

The date on your certification or how many years you've been on the job has no bearing on how well you perform your job.

Nothing conducive to life ever follows the uttering of "Oh shit!"

When talking to management, much like talking to your girlfriend or boyfriend, nothing good ever follows "We need to talk."

Something good *always* follows "See, right. What happened was..."

Contrary to popular belief, talking slowly, loudly, and with exaggerated mouth movements *does not* help bridge the language barrier.

Similarly, adding "O" to the end of words is not speaking Spanish.

Arrive alive; don't let the part timer drive.

When someone says, "It hurts when I do this," the motion that follows *never* serves any discernable function in life.

The life you save could take your own.

CPR is not a summer sport.

No matter what time you set shift change for, someone will inevitably call for an ambulance at that time.

Similarly, no matter what time you sit down to eat, some-one will call for an ambulance. When you ask them when their problem started, it will always be several hours *before* you sat down to eat.

Clear plastic wrap is apparently an acceptable and safe substitution for a broken windshield on your car. If you want tinted windows, use a black garbage bag... *(Please don't.)*

Clearly, hiding your alcohol in a brown paper bag will fool *anyone* into thinking there is nothing illegal in there.

I'd rather be paid poorly doing a job I love than be paid highly for a job I can't stand.

THINGS YOU NEVER WANT TO HEAR YOUR RESCUER SAY

"Oops!"

"Holy shit!"

"The book never told me about *that!*"

"Honestly, I know what I'm doing; I'm just having an off day."

"Wow, what do you know? The book *was* right."

"I'm sorry, what were you saying? I wasn't paying attention."

"No, don't worry. I'm not laughing *at* you."

"Is your family coming with us? No? Good."

"I've never seen *that* before."

"That's not supposed to happen."

"That's not good."

"That's fucking cool!"

"I guess that will have to do."

"Does your heart always do that?"

"Why do they come to me to die?"

"Ah, gees, not again!"

"Anyone see where I put my... Oh, no."

"Oh, the guys back at the station are gonna love this."

"Walk towards the light, old friend."

"Well, I'm stumped!"

"You *really* should have told me *that* sooner."

"Do you want to say goodbye to your family?"

"Didn't old Mrs. Smith do that right before she... forget I said anything."

"You want to go to what hospital? Oh no, they could never handle *this*."

"Please don't sit so close."

"What on earth is that smell?"

"Man, that had to hurt!"

"Wallet? What wallet?"

"Does this hurt? No? It *should.*"

"That's okay, I hear voices too."

"Aw, I understand. I can't afford my medications either."

"Whoa, don't touch me!"

"Did you ever have a heart attack *before* today?"

ODD DISPATCHES

I was dispatched to a possible baby delivery in progress at an infertility clinic. Luckily I didn't have to assist in the delivery, but being dispatched to an infertility clinic for an imminent birth seems like one heck of an oxymoron to me.

I heard an ambulance dispatched to a doctor's office for a "sick person." I'm sorry, isn't that the point of a doctor's office? What's next, a dentist office for a toothache?

I was dispatched to a person's home for a toothache one night. The patient said he wanted to go to a particular hospital because it had a dental clinic. He had the nerve to argue with me when I told him it was only open during daytime business hours. He was under the impression that the hospital would simply call in a dentist for his toothache at 11pm. Upon hearing this, the nurse in the ER made him wait until the clinic opened, at 9am.

I was dispatched to the parking lot of a hospital for an unconscious patient. I understand it is technically illegal for ER staff to help someone outside of the ER because of bureaucratic bullshit, but was it too much to ask that someone get the patient inside?

A friend was dispatched to a funeral home for a cardiac arrest. I know it was a grieving family member who went into cardiac arrest, but for a moment, I feared that someone who was in denial called 911 for the body in the casket.

Stranger things have happened.

Another friend was dispatched to a funeral home for a dead body. The hospital had given the wrong body to the funeral home when they came to pick it up. The funeral home staff was about to embalm it when they realized it was the wrong body. Rather than bring it back, they called an ambulance.

I was dispatched to a chocolate factory for a diabetic emergency. *Makes you wonder what came first, employment at the factory or the diabetes?*

I was dispatched for a dead body in a cemetery. It was an overdose a few days old, but you can imagine what was going through my mind as I responded.

My rescue squad was dispatched to a parking lot for a motor vehicle accident with a rollover. *How does one roll over a car going 5 miles per hour?*

I heard an ambulance dispatched to a movie theater for a violent emotionally disturbed person. I know you're thinking the same thing I was – what movie was it and was it *that* good to drive someone into an insane rage?

The movie was *Bordello of Blood*. Be your own judge of that.

I was dispatched to look for a naked man running through traffic, holding a can of tuna. I see two things wrong with this:

1. Why would someone look close enough at a naked person running through traffic to see that he was holding a can of tuna?

2. Why did they feel it was important to point out that the person was holding a can of anything? Were they afraid I would pick up the *wrong* naked man running through traffic?

Alas, I never found my naked guy; the police transported him to the hospital before we got there. As for the tuna…

Similarly, I heard an ambulance dispatched to a shopping mall for "a possible emotionally disturbed person, walking around in front of *The Children's Place*, wearing a hospital robe."

First off, what makes him emotionally disturbed just because he's wearing a hospital gown? It was over a hundred degrees that day; maybe he was trying to keep cool. I would wear a hospital gown if I had the butt for it.

Secondly, how was he able to make it all the way to the mall without someone calling sooner? It was a far walk from any area hospital. Can you imagine the uncomfortable looks on the faces of the people he rode the bus with?

One night I was quite surprised to hear that the asthmatic patient one paramedic unit was sent for was actually a shooting. How the 911 operator can get "I'm having an asthma attack" out of "I've been shot" still escapes me.

DEALING WITH DANGEROUS SCENES

Not many people think of EMS as a dangerous occupation. Sure they recognize the fact that driving is a dangerous aspect of the job, as well as dealing with contagious diseases. However, many people are shocked that I have been attacked by patients. A sad fact of the job is that we routinely walk unsuspectingly into dangerous scenes. Many times, a scene is safe one minute, then something unseen or out of our control will instantly change things.

Some EMTs and paramedics wear bulletproof vests. It's not that shocking when you think about how we look entering a scene. We have lights and sirens; the police have lights and sirens. We wear uniforms; the police wear uniforms. Some of us wear badges; so do the police. At first glance, we may look like police at a scene. In New York City, the police and Fire/EMS personnel all wear the same color uniforms. The only way to tell them apart is by the big logos on the back of the shirts – NYPD or FDNY.

Do I wear a vest? On occasion. When I know there is heavy alcohol intake on that night or a potential for violence, I do. I always wear one on Christmas, New Year's, and the night before Halloween. I hate wearing them because they are uncomfortable as hell. I don't feel any safer in them either. I figure a person is more likely to beat my ass or stab me than they are to shoot me. But I have, on occasions, been shot at and had guns pulled on me.

I was dispatched for a shooting in front of a police station. I approached the scene cautiously, and saw multiple police officers surrounding the scene. I turned off the lights as I normally do and was waved into the scene by officers. I figured the scene was secured and proceeded in.

I got set to treat my patient when I heard two or three pops. My partner looked at me with alarm. Being from the quiet suburbs, I had no idea what that sound was. I heard several more pops. Then the window of the car next to me shattered. At that point, I believe my partner and I wet our pants and dove on the ground screaming like little children. *Okay, so I'm exaggerating a wee bit.*

An ambulance was dispatched to a shooting outside of a bar. They waited several minutes for a police car, then decided to enter the area to see what was going on.

Two men were lying on the ground bleeding from several bullet wounds. A few people stood around staring in awe at what had happened. The crew decided to move quickly. They called for another ambulance and began treating both men.

One EMT was treating the more serious of the two men – two gunshot wounds in his abdomen and one in his chest. So engrossed in what he was doing, he almost didn't hear the clicking sound behind him. Then a calm voice said to him, "I meant to kill him. I didn't mean to hurt the other guy. Help the other guy." The EMT turned around to see the shooter pointing the gun at his head.

That is why we don't enter the scene without police on shooting calls. I can't say anything bad about the EMTs on that call; we've all done it. There aren't many feelings in the world worse than being capable of helping someone, but not able to get to them.

However, danger from firearms is not just a danger at the scene of a shooting.

I was dispatched to assist one of our regular patients in an apartment building. She was a nice old lady and had been sick for several days. *No biggie, I love calls like that.* Usually they just need to see a private doctor and can walk to the ambulance. I thought this was going to be a routine run. *Wrong!*

As we were getting ready to load her, someone began pounding on the front door screaming something in Spanish. Through my amazing mastery of the Spanish language (*note the sarcasm*), I was able to decipher that she needed an ambulance. *The fact that she was screaming 'Ambulancia!' gave that away; anything beyond that was lost on me.*

I opened the door and this woman in the hallway began screaming at the top of her lungs that she needed help. *I don't know why people continue to scream once they already have my attention.* I asked her to calm down while I tried to call my dispatcher and let him know I needed another ambulance. She would not stop screaming.

And my biggest problem in all this is that I talk so low on the radio. I speak in a normal conversational tone so that I'm not screaming in the dispatcher's ear. I've been doing it so long that it just comes natural to me. So as I was trying to talk, all my dispatcher was hearing was this lady screaming.

He thinks she's me and that I'm getting attacked (*Although I take offense to that because I don't scream like a girl... not usually anyway.*) and he calls for the cavalry. So every ambulance and paramedic unit in the city came rushing to my aid. Because of the construction of the building, I couldn't transmit a clear message to tell them I was okay. It was a pretty good thing I couldn't.

Finally I managed to yell loud enough for her to "shut the fuck up" and asked her to speak English, which she was able to do perfectly. *Which is another point that is completely lost on me. We live in America. In America we speak English. So if you know English, why not speak it when you need help? The chance is very good the person coming to help you speaks English.* She told me that her brother had been beaten up.

I looked in the apartment and saw a young man sitting on the couch holding a towel on his head. I told her to stay outside while I went to treat him. She said okay and stood in the hallway. I asked him what happened and he told me that he got into a fight with a group of guys because one of the guys had gotten his thirteen-year old sister pregnant. *Wonderful dynamic here, these guys were all over twenty-four.* They hit him in the head with a bottle and that was the end of the fight.

I looked at his head. It wasn't too serious, but I thought it would probably need a couple of stitches. "Do I have to go?" He asked me.

"You don't have to do anything you don't want to, but I think you should go and get looked at." With that, the lady (I still have no idea who she was.), came running back into the room screaming her head off.

"Why do you think I should go?"

I always try to be honest with my patients, but this was a time when I should have made up some bullshit. "You may need a few stitches." Even as the words flew out of my mouth, I knew they were the wrong words to say.

"Stitches? Motherfucker, it's on now!"

I didn't know what *it* he was referring to, but I knew it couldn't be good. He got up, pushed past me and stormed into his bedroom. I knew I probably shouldn't have followed him, but it was like I was on autopilot. Stupid me tried to calmly tell him it wasn't that bad, which it wasn't. But the bandage had fallen off his head and he saw the blood trickling down his face when he looked in the mirror.

He sat on his bed and I thought I had made a break-through. Then he reached under his mattress and pulled out a gun. "Get the fuck out of my way," he ordered and aimed the gun at my head. He could have easily pushed by me, but instead he held me at gunpoint. For what seemed like hours, but was only seconds, the only sound I could hear was my heart racing.

I tried to remain calm, thinking what would Robert De Niro do in a situation like this: come up with a witty line and a killer delivery for it, then crack the bastard's skull open and say something even cooler as he beat the snot out of the guy... *Okay, so De Niro was out of the question.*

So I did what most people would have done – I babbled uncontrollably.

"Hey buddy," I stammered, "you don't want that to get infected, do you?" He continued to say nothing with the gun to my head. "We'll get you fixed up and then you can do whatever you want to do." In my mind I couldn't believe I was talking about infections with a guy with a gun to my head. *What was next? Hey buddy, you know a nasty infection will only throw off your aim?*

"What good is shooting me if your head just gets infected and you die anyway?"

He paused and began thinking about what I said. "I'll take you to the hospital, get ya stitched up, and then anything you want to do is *your* own business. I don't know nothing, I don't want to know nothing. Sound good?"

He nodded and stashed the gun under the bed. He gave me a suspicious look and I think I read his mind. I looked toward the mattress and said, "I didn't see a thing." He flashed a smile at me and I realized we were cool and it was over. *One final blast of nervous gas from my ass and I was ready to rock and roll.*

Just when I was about to get him up and out of the room, the cavalry showed up. I turned around to find at least twelve co-workers cramming into this tiny apartment. They rushed into the bedroom and sat him down on the bed to start examining him. The lady from the hallway followed them in and began screaming again. "Tell ya what guys, let's do this outside," I said to the one who seemed to have taken the lead.

"No, we can do it here."

"No," I said, trying to be inconspicuous. "I think you want to do this outside."

"Why? We can do it here."

I pulled him aside and said, "Because she's a nut and he's got a piece under the bed."

After a momentary pause, the EMT flashed me a smile. "Well, Mr. Kerins, I concur with your assessment. Let's convene this outside."

A friend of mine was dispatched to an apartment complex in the city for one of the most routine of calls, a baby with a fever. As he walked through the parking lot toward the building, they began receiving gunfire. A man had stabbed his girlfriend in another apartment and began shooting when he saw the flashing lights.

An ambulance and EMS supervisor responded for a suicidal man who subsequently barricaded himself inside his house when they knocked on the door. He yelled at the supervisor that he had a gun and he would shoot if he heard any cops coming. The supervisor tried her best to calm him down. Unfortunately she was unaware of other events just down the street.

A group of gunmen shot up and robbed an armored car. Responding police officers were on a course that led directly outside the man's window. As they flew by, sirens wailing, to assist the shooting victims at the robbery, the EDP became scared they were coming for him. He immediately began blasting wildly through the door at the crew.

No EMS personnel were injured, but after an extremely long stand- off, the EDP shot himself in the stomach.

My brother did some of his paramedic training time in Jersey City a few years before I began working there. He ran into some trouble with the Latin Kings street gang after the Dominican Day Parade. The EMTs were responding to a call and got into a brawl with a group of Kings after some words were passed. His partner hit the panic button and help was on the way.

Salvation came over a PA system. An ambulance that was close by, and staffed by two very proud Irish men, came barreling over the hill blasting bagpipe music over the loudspeaker. The Kings dropped everything and ran away.

I was dispatched for a "non-violent" emotionally disturbed person waiting for us on the corner. Because the person was "non violent," we saw no need to wait for the police.

When we arrived on scene, the police were there already anyway, about four cars. I didn't think much of it. We saw some officers walking into an abandoned wooded lot and for some reason thought it would be a good idea to follow them.

An officer came stumbling out of the woods to meet us. "Listen guys, we can't find him, but if you see him, *don't go near him!*"

That never sounds promising. *Ok, I'll bite,* "Why not?"

"He just escaped from the Psychiatric ER and was running loose on Ocean Ave beating people with a fence post."

Who screens these calls?

Right after that we were dispatched to the eleventh floor of a housing project for a "non-violent" EDP. *You would think we'd have learned from the previous episode, but then I wouldn't have material for a sequel.*

We rode the elevator to the eleventh floor and were just about to knock on the door when someone screamed something about the ambulance in Spanish. I don't know what they said, but it couldn't have been good when it was followed with "Shut the fuck up or I'll fucking kill you!" So rather than see what was waiting for us on the other side of the door, we decided to retreat back downstairs and wait for the police.

We pressed the button for the elevator and waited an eternity for it. I started whistling *The Girl from Ipanema* and other elevator music standards as we waited. Before the elevator could reach the floor, a large crash and more yelling about the ambulance came from the patient's room. With that my partner and I looked at each other and both said, "Stairs!"

We ran down the hall in a panic. My partner kicked open a door and ran into the dark room. "Dave!" I screamed.

"What?"

"That's the broom closet!"

"How do you know?"

"There's a sign!" I pointed to the sign that clearly stated broom closet.

He ran out with a stupid grin on his face. We paused for a minute, then there was more fighting from in the apartment. I grabbed him and we ran for what we were sure were the stairs.

Normal, rational people would probably have run down a flight or two and gotten on the elevator there. Not me, not us! *No siree!* We thought it would be the wisest move to run down all eleven floors. But the fifth floor I was so dizzy I missed the handrail and took a header down the stairs.

I was dispatched for a patient having a seizure. We were told that it was a potentially unsafe scene, and not to enter without the police. Normal procedure is to park the truck in such a position that allows us to see if police have arrived but not so the people in the house can see us. I don't know what my partner was thinking, but we parked in a pretty obvious spot. We sat there for a few minutes waiting for the police. As I called our dispatcher to try to get an ETA for the police, someone ran out of the apartment building and approached the ambulance. Before my partner had a chance to throw the truck into drive, the guy was at our window pounding on it.

"Why aren't you helping us?"

Without rolling down the window, my partner yelled, "Because someone's being violent in the apartment and we were told to wait for the police."

"Nobody's being violent, we were just yelling at that dumb bitch on the phone because she was asking us too many questions."

I probably should have stood my ground, but I have no idea what I was thinking. "Listen, you tell your family. The first one who yells at me, I'm out the door. You understand?"

The guy nodded and ran upstairs. He quickly ran back downstairs and said everyone would be okay. Still, I cautiously approached the upstairs apartment. Everyone inside was calm and grateful to see the ambulance. The patient, a fairly large man, was lying on his back on the floor in his boxer shorts.

"What happened?"

The patient's mother answered, "He had a seizure." The patient appeared to be post-ictal, so it was conceivable that he had seizure. He was flopping around on the floor, talking like a three-year old. However, through further questioning, I found out that the patient had allegedly had a seizure over an hour ago and walked home. *That doesn't sound like a seizure, but it was three in the morning and I didn't feel like arguing.*

Normally I would have cancelled the paramedics who were coming. It didn't seem like a seizure, more like this guy was drunk or on drugs. However, I kept them coming because I knew I would need the help lifting him if he couldn't walk. It's a very good thing I didn't cancel them.

After a few minutes of waiting for the patient to come around with the oxygen, we decided it wasn't working and we would have to lift him downstairs. The second we touched him to try to get him onto the Reeves, he swung at my partner. My partner instinctively grabbed his arm and didn't let go. The patient tried to swing his other arm, so one of the medics grabbed that one. He started kicking around and I dove on his legs.

Before someone starts thinking we're trying to beat our patient, I must explain. At this point, we have to first prevent injury to ourselves, then calm the patient down. If any of us were to let up, this big man would have definitely injured one or more of us. I made it a point to explain this to the family. They seemed angry at first because they thought we were trying to hurt him. Once I explained to them the necessity of what we were doing, they understood and were on our side.

We needed a little more help to carry the combative patient down the stairs. I keyed up my radio and calmly call for an addition ambulance. Much to my horror, I saw that the brand new paramedic was screaming into the radio for help. Apparently he had never been presented with a situation like this before. I tried to call the dispatcher to tell everyone to relax, but it was too late. A citywide assist had been called, and everyone was hurrying to my aid because it sounded like this guy was killing us. Within minutes, the small room our patient was in was filled with EMS uniforms. Some many people were in the room that people had to stand on furniture.

This was an example of how things can get out of control very quickly. Most of the assisting units were helping to restrain the patient. Others were standing by with equipment and moving furniture to try to make it easier to get through the apartment. One person, however, took it upon himself to yell at and berate the family members. I got up to try to stop him.

He was yelling at the patient's brother and sister. I have no idea why; they weren't in the way and were actually on our side. As I made my way over to settle the dispute, I noticed that the tattoos on the man he was yelling at matched the tattoos on the patient and the tattoos on the friend in the hallway. I couldn't help but notice that these tattoos all matched the tattoos of Latin King gang members. At the same moment I made that recognition, I heard the brother yell, "That's it, fuck this motherfucka! I'm getting my shit!"

I don't know what his "shit" was, but it couldn't be good when it was preceded by the phrase, "fuck this motherfucka!" In what felt like 'super slow motion,' I dove across the room, *Noooooooooooooooooooooooo!*

It was time for "Super Nice Devin." I don't like my alter ego, because it uses way too much energy to be that nice. But I had to settle this before the entire team got shot. I threw the EMT out of the apartment and was able to settle things with the brother, sister, and other gang members.

We were able to move the patient downstairs and get him to the hospital. And after all that wrestling with the patient, all the arguing with the family, and all my hard work as Super Nice Devin, the patient walked out of the hospital before I had a chance to finish my paperwork.

That felt like a complete waste of energy.

KENNEDY BOULEVARD AND SEAVIEW DRIVE

01:25 hours

Things seem to have returned to normal, if there is a "normal." My truck smells pine fresh and has a shine to it that might win an award at a parade. I'm comfortable that all of the nasty funk we'd accumulated tonight has been wiped completely away. It's time to start anew, and more importantly, to catch some shut-eye.

Sleep will come shortly, I hope. My partner has pulled over at this intersection so he can run into his girlfriend's house for a clean uniform shirt and something to drink. *At least that's what he tells me...*

For some reason, I don't feel comfortable falling asleep right here. I decide it's probably best to hold off napping until my partner returns. Instead, I pick up the Tom Clancy novel I've been reading at work and get lost in the action. I roll the window up and crank up the air conditioner. It's not that hot any more, but I can relax better when it's cold. I'm deep into the story. The Soviet army has just invaded Iceland, and as tired as I am, I can't put the book down. Suddenly, there is a banging at my window.

You've got to be kidding me! Isn't it too late for this bullshit?

An eerie sense of *deja vu* over takes me as I see a man in his thirties swaying back and forth as he looks into my window. *Can't drunks leave me alone for one night?* He's making the universal sign for 'roll your window down.' As he does so, his body rocks back and forth.

Very reluctantly, I roll down my window. "Can I help you?"

The man looks up and down the street, as if trying to find the right words to say. I follow his gaze as he looks up Kennedy Blvd and down it, as if maybe there's something I'm missing. Finally, he takes a deep breath, steadies himself, and speaks. "Do you know where the number ten bus stops?"

Do I look like I know where the number ten bus stops?

"No sir, I don't. Good night." I abruptly roll up my window. I pick where I left off, with the Marines trying to hide from the invading Soviets. I get that feeling like I'm being watched, and slowly I turn my head to look out my window. Not surprisingly, he's still there.

He smiles at me, then makes that universal sign again. More reluctantly, and extremely pissed off, I roll down my window. "What?"

"You work for the city, right?"

Where is this going? "Yeah."

"Then my taxes pay your salary, right?"

"What the hell do you want?"

"Well, see," his speech is extremely slurred, "the way I look at it, since I pay your salary, you can give me a ride home."

"Yeah, you see it that way? That's not how it is. Now please go away." I roll up the window again. No sooner do I turn my head to look at my book, than there is a thumping on the window. Now I'm pissed, *really pissed*. I'm not usually confrontational, but I've tried to be nice and it's gotten me nowhere. Intimidation time? *Okay, so we know that won't work, but we can try.*

I step out of the truck and slam the door. "What do you want now?"

He staggers backwards, and then begins looking around for the right words to say. "I live by City General. Can't you just drop me off?"

"Are you still at this? I am not a taxi! Now unless you're sick, leave me the hell alone!"

I should really think about what I say before it exits my lips.

He looks at me a moment longer, then grabs his head. "I have a headache. You should take me to the hospital."

"Stop fucking around! There are genuinely sick people out there and I don't have time to waste with you!"

"But I asked for an ambulance. Now you have to take me."

Damn, out on a technicality! Won't someone please *change that law!*

"Three-Oh-Nine to dispatch," I call in. "We've been flagged down at the Boulevard and Seaview for an intoxicated person."

Frustrated, I open the back door. "Get in." He stumbles his way into the back. He begins to sit down in the captain's chair. "No!" I yell, "That's my chair! Sit here!" Roughly, I guide his hips so he flops down on the bench seat.

"Aw, thanks, mister." He extends his hand to offer me a handshake. I brusquely push it away.

"Shut up."

"Why do you have to be so rude?"

"Why? Because you're wasting my time! And when you waste my time, someone dies!"

"Aw, I'm sorry. But thanks, mister."

He's still jovial. Why? Haven't I been rotten enough to him? I need to work on being rude. Apparently the only person I can piss off to the point she doesn't want to talk to me any more is my girlfriend.

My partner comes trotting back to the ambulance. "What's going on?" He pops his head into the truck and laughs. "Can't I leave you alone for five minutes?"

"Apparently not."

"Where does he want to go?"

"City General, but aren't they on divert?"

"I don't think so." I shot him a look and he catches on to what I'm saying. "Oh yeah, that's right."

I'm not about to let this bum beat me.

"What's going on?" The patient asks.

"We can't take you to City General," my partner explains, "because they're not accepting patients."

"Well, that's okay," he says, "I don't really need to be seen. I just want to be dropped off closer to my house."

"Look you, either you're a patient or you're not. If you are, you go to a hospital that can treat you. If not, you get the fuck out of my bus!"

"Okay," he says reluctantly, "I'll go to another hospital. What's closest to City General?"

Excellent, he's playing right into my trap!

"City South is right around the corner."

"Fine, take me there."

It's actually a short ride to City South Hospital, but it seems torturously long as I try to keep from exploding on this babbling drunken fool. He refuses to shut up, annoying me with questions about my job, and apologies for 'wasting' my time. My partner opens the door and guides the man out so that he doesn't fall on his face. *What a tragedy that would be!*

I grab his other arm and hustle him into the ER. I find an empty bed and nudge him onto it. "Thanks guys," he calls out as I walk away.

"Why did you bring him here?" The nurse asks.

"Because of your particular way of dealing with drunks."

The nurse and my partner shake their heads. "You're wrong," my partner says as he washes his hands.

The nurse smiles. "I'll get the Foley."

Every drunk that we bring into City South gets a Foley Catheter. If you don't know what that is, look it up.

Game, set, match!

UNCONSCIOUS, INTOXICATED, AND/OR EXPIRED

Once, around Halloween, we were called to an abandoned lot for a "man down." When we arrived, all we found was a heavily wooded lot. We attempted to enter, only to see a half a dozen junkies go running off into the woods. We decided the risk was entirely too great to go without police, so we waited. A man on a bicycle came rolling down the street yelling to us, "Did you find him?" When we said no, he offered to show us where the patient was.

Being that is was getting close to the end of my shift and I had been working for twenty-four hours straight, I did not feel like waiting around for the police, we followed the man. Seventy-five yards into the woods, and covered by thick brush, we found the patient. I turned to the caller and said what was the burning question on everyone's mind, "How the fuck did you expect us to find him?"

The patient was blue and covered in his own wastes. We rapidly evacuated him to the street. However, in the process, I got his excrement on my pants – *as if I wasn't pissed enough to begin with.* Now it was time for some payback. I am a petty man, and not afraid to admit it.

DEVIN KERINS | 159

The paramedics started the IV, and began administering the Narcan to reverse the heroin while I set the scene. We turned off the lights in the back of the truck, except for the medic's MagLite. I put three-inch tape across his eye brows. When he started to stir like the Narcan was kicking in, I yanked the tape off his eyes. He woke up screaming. The medic leaned over him with the flashlight on his face and vampire fangs in his mouth and began hissing. The patient screamed again and let loose his bowels once more.

On the 2000 Fourth of July weekend, I had to work at OpSail, a large gathering of ships from militaries and private owners around the world. During the weekend before, I was on duty in the park when someone's friend overdosed on a large amount of heroin. His friend, looking out for the patient, tried to dump him in front of the State Police Field Headquarters in the park and get away.

When I arrived, the State Troopers had him at gunpoint and the patient was convulsing on the ground. We threw the patient in the ambulance and immediately began working on him. A Trooper opened the door and asked me to go through the patient's pockets to see if he had any paraphernalia on him. I said absolutely not because that isn't part of my job, but not wanting to interfere with the State Police, I came up with a better solution. I cut the patient's pants off and handed them to the Trooper. "What happens when he wakes up?" He asked.

I grabbed a tube of SurgiLube and dumped a giant glob down the back of his underwear. When the patient came too, instead of fighting like heroin overdoses usually do, he bolted upright and cried, "Where are my pants?" His next question: "Why is my ass wet?"

"Maybe next time you shouldn't do heroin around strangers," I replied.

"What does that mean?"

"Does your ass hurt?"

"No."

"Good," I said calmly and went about my paperwork.

He broke down into tears and wailed, "What did they do to me?"

I hope this will be enough to get him to stop doing heroin, but probably not.

I thought I was bad, but I met my idol. A medic in Philadelphia had an interesting way of having fun with overdoses: he would remove one of their shoes. Why? Well, when they woke up they would be faced with the dilemma of trying to figure out where the other shoe went. When they couldn't figure that out, they would have to make the decision of what to do about it.

They could throw the remaining shoe away. But then what would they do if they found the missing one?

They could keep it in hopes of finding the new shoe. But what if they never found it?

The other medics said they could always tell this medic's patients because they would be walking out of the hospital with disappointed looks on their faces and only one shoe on.

I responded for an "unconscious" to a building that houses several government offices. On the way in, we attracted the stares of several interested onlookers. All they did was stare; no one bothered to hold to door for us. I double-checked my pager and made sure the office we wanted was on the third floor. I grabbed the first gawker and asked, "Do you know where the elevator is?"

"What? The deliverer? Oh shit! Someone's having a baby! Hey everyone, someone's having a baby!"

It wasn't bad enough that he completely misunderstood me, but everyone began crowding in front of us to look at our empty stretcher, preventing me from rapidly accessing my unconscious patient who was now allegedly delivering a baby.

I should consider a second career in public relations.

I was dispatched for a fall one night. The mother of the child who fell apologized to me the whole way to the hospital because she felt she was "wasting" our time because her child wasn't that seriously hurt. I tried my best to assure her that she really wasn't wasting my time. She was so impressed by how nice we were that she wanted my supervisor's name so she could write a nice thank you letter.

As soon as I gave her his name, we heard there was a shooting around the corner from the hospital we were at. The nice Mr. Kerins suddenly changed when we arrived on scene. The police were calling for us to put a rush on our response, so I parked the truck in the middle of the street, tying up traffic, got out, and ran for the building. Someone got out of their car and started yelling at me to move the truck, which elicited the usual response: "Fuck off!"

I ran up the three flights of stairs faster than I usually like to move and pressed my way past several police officers and paused at the door to catch my breath. A young man had tragically shot himself in the head after an argument with family. I was about to call it in as a DOA, when a lady in the room started yelling at us. She was in nurse's scrubs and sitting on the edge of the bed, holding the man's head.

"Get in here and do something!"

Normally there is not much to do when someone shoots himself in the head. If done right, his brain is destroyed by the cavitation of the bullet and even if we could save him, he would be on a ventilator for the rest of his life. Figuring she was related, I tried to be nice. "Ma'am, please step away."

"No! You get in here and do something!"

That's when I noticed the gun was still next to him. Now

she could potentially shoot herself or one of us by accident, so I needed to get her away. "Ma'am, please get away from there."

"No! Get in here and do something now!"

"Step away from the body."

"I don't have to listen to you! Do you know who I am?"

"No! Who are you?"

"I'm an operating room nurse."

"That's great. Now get away."

"I know what I'm doing!"

I couldn't believe I was having a shouting match over a dead body. But I was rapidly losing my temper. "When was the last time someone blew their brains out in the OR?"

"Don't talk to me like that! I'm holding pressure on the injury."

The injury pattern looked like he actually placed the gun in his mouth and shot through the roof of his mouth and out the back of his head, and she was holding 'pressure' on his jaw. *Translation: she was doing nothing!* Seeing I was getting nowhere, I turned my attention to the police. "Look, secure the gun."

The officer bent over to get the gun and the lady swung at him and started yelling, "Get away. They need to do something!" The officers began yelling at her. Suddenly everyone in the room was yelling and my head was about to explode.

"Everyone SHUT UP!" My sudden break from sanity managed to quiet the room. "Now, ma'am, I've tried to be nice. You need to get out... *now!*"

"I don't have to listen to you, you're just an EMT. I am a nurse."

That did it. I lost it. "You need to shut the fuck up and get the fuck out so I can do what I need to do!"

That stunned her long enough for two officers to grab her and yank her from the room. The patient still had a pulse, but was not breathing. That upset me because now I had to work on the patient. I know that sounds insensitive, but I knew I would be wasting my effort for no reason at all; he was gone no matter what. After vigorous efforts to save him, the patient was finally pronounced at the ER.

The lady, who we still don't know if she was related or not, later waved down my supervisor while he was responding to another call and apologized for her behavior.

Dispatched for a respiratory distress patient one morning, I arrived at the senior citizens' high-rise to find my patient clinging to the air conditioner unit, desperately trying to breathe. He had several young family members sitting around the room, looking completely disinterested in what was going on. I found this odd for a moment because it seemed too early in the morning for his family members to be visiting, but I didn't think much of it and continued on with my assessment.

I quickly ruled out asthma and pulmonary edema because his lung sounds were clear. I did a little further digging and found out that all of this started when he woke up and was paranoid and thinking about dead relatives. *So he's having an anxiety attack,* no big deal. We helped him down to the ambulance and started taking him over to the hospital. Half way to the hospital, the patient turned to me and said, "Can I ask you something?"

Usually something good follows that statement.

"Sure, go ahead."

"Okay, hypothetically, say my family were smoking crack cocaine when I was asleep, might it cause this?"

"Are you asking this hypothetically, or are you sure they smoke crack in your house?"

"No, they smoke crack in my house."

"Sir, you're eighty years old! It can't *possibly* be good for you to be smoking crack!"

"Well, I'm not smoking it!"

Do you think it's possible for the Surgeon General to put warnings on the side of crack rocks about the effects of secondhand crack smoke?

I responded for a "man down." When I arrived, we found our patient slumped over against the side of someone's house. He wasn't moving and lay with his arm slung across his chest.

"Think that's our patient?" My partner said sarcastically.

"Think he's drunk?"

I quipped back, "Either that or he's dead."

The patient began crying, "No mister. Don't leave me. I'm not dead yet!"

A paramedic crew was working on a man who was having chest pain and going in and out of consciousness. When they hooked him up to the heart monitor, they saw his heart was in ventricular tachycardia (V-Tach). *For the cardiology illiterate out there,* definitely *not a good thing.* Overall, he was going downhill fast—they would have to shock his heart back into a normal, life sustaining rhythm.

They set up the pads to shock him, and before they could do anything, he went unconscious. They immediately shocked him and he went into a normal rhythm. They gave him the appropriate follow up medications and started transporting to the hospital.

En route, he went unconscious and back into V-Tach. This time, he had no pulses with the V-Tach. They shocked him again, and he converted to a normal rhythm once more. As they pulled up to the ER, he went into a pulseless V-Tach once more. They shocked him and he converted again. *At least he's being consistent.*

When they transferred him over to the ER bed, the nurse yelled out that he had gone into V-Tach once more. Not bothering to check for a pulse or if he was even conscious or not, she shocked him again.

The noise in the ER was silenced by the man's cry, "Owww! You motherfuckers!" *360 joules of electricity can really hurt someone if they're awake to feel it!*

I responded to an "altered mental status" and found the patient going in and out of consciousness. We placed her on the heart monitor and found her to be in a supraventricular tachycardia. Basically, her heart was beating entirely too fast. We needed to move fast. Ideally, we would have liked to start an IV and give her some sedation for what we were about to do. Unfortunately, she had horrible veins.

We had to cardiovert her – send 100 joules of electricity into her to slow her heart rate down. I've never been cardioverted, but I can't imagine that's a pleasant feeling. She didn't speak any English, and the most Spanish my partner could come up with was *"Mucho dolor ahora!"* She shot a quick, scared look at us just as he pushed the shock button.

There was the usual *thump*, she jumped, and screamed "Please God! Don't do that again! I'm begging you."

I stood there in amazement. "Dude," I said, "we shocked English into her!"

An ambulance was dispatched to a nursing home for an unresponsive patient. When they arrived, the patient was seated, motionless, with his eyes open. The EMTs felt something was wrong as they approached the patient. He didn't look like he was breathing. One EMT felt for a pulse and found none.

"When was the last time someone talked to him?"

"Ah, this morning at shift change."

The EMT went on to check if there was rigor mortis in the jaw. The jaw was stiff and cold. Something caught the EMT's attention, and he took out a pair of forceps. Out of the mouth he pulled a large chunk of Salisbury steak. He dropped it on the tray in front of the patient and something else caught his eye. It was the menu for the week. Salisbury steak was on the menu *two* days ago. *Shift change, my ass! He'd been dead for almost 48 hours.*

I was dispatched to a familiar address for an unconscious diabetic female. I had known the family for years. I used to take the wife in for dialysis. I mentioned to my partner while we were responding that this had to be legitimate because the husband was very responsible and that he never called for us unless it was truly necessary.

The BLS arrived before us and were on scene for what seemed like an unusually long time for this particular crew. That meant they were either obtaining a refusal from the patient or that the patient was critical and they were really working up there. We met up with them as they were coming downstairs. One look at the patient and I knew this was legitimate. She was still unconscious, sweating, and breathing erratically. We immediately began working on her and sped to the hospital.

One of the EMTs looked at me shaking her head. "You'll never guess what happened. The husband said she was becoming combative and altered mental status. He figured it was her sugar, so he duct taped her to a wheelchair and gave her a shot of insulin."

(For those not familiar with Diabetic emergencies, a patient begins acting like that when their sugar becomes low. Insulin is given to bring down the sugar levels in the blood. So if you gave insulin to someone whose sugar was low already, you basically wipe out any sugar they have left... not a good thing!)

I guess I was wrong about the husband.

FOR ANIMAL LOVERS

I responded for an unconscious, possible cardiac arrest. A lady was waiting outside for us, waving us down. We followed her upstairs and I heard a dog barking. "Ma'am, can you please lock the dog up?"

"I already took care of him."

Okay, can we guess what the first thing I saw was when I opened up the door? *A pit bull!* "Ma'am, can you *please* lock the dog up." As I said that, I noticed there was a cat next to the dog.

I am *very* allergic to cats.

"Ma'am, can you also lock up the cat."

"Oh, I can't handle all them cats," she said.

"All them cats?" I asked. I opened the door and saw not one, not two, but *thirteen* cats. All of these balls of allergens were crawling over my unconscious patient.

I saw my patient was blue and not breathing, so I figured it would be a cut and dry pronouncement. I held my breath and ran past all the cats to check for a pulse. My patient was sprawled out on the bathroom floor and looked dead. I reached down to feel for a pulse and she gasped for air. She scared the heck out of me. I screamed some choice words and fell back onto two of the cats. The patient was given the heroin antidote and walked out of the ER a few minutes after we brought her in, but *I* spent the rest of the afternoon hooked up to heart monitors in the emergency room.

I responded to an unconscious patient. When I arrived, the EMTs were running out of the house gagging. That usually means the person has been dead so long that the decomposition has become so extensive it turns the stomach. You can think of that as a bad thing, but from the standpoint of a busy paramedic, it's a good thing. *Less paperwork!*

You can imagine my dismay when I asked the EMTs what they had seen and they said, "She's still alive!" Now my mind wondered what could be so bad that they were gagging.

My partner and I decided it was up to us to make sense of this situation and rapidly get the patient out. As we walked inside, the smell became tangible. The air had a certain thickness that made it harder to breathe, in spite of the stench, an overpowering mix of feces, mildew, rotting milk, cigarettes, dust, fish, onions, and something that I couldn't quite put my finger on just yet.

As I entered the front door with the Reeves stretcher, one of the EMTs handed me a surgical mask and a bottle of Vicks rub she had confiscated from a neighbor. I had to give her a pat on the back for that thought. "All right, let's go," I said to her as I motioned inside.

"No way! I'm not going in there!" Rather than argue with her, I chalked it up to her usual laziness and walked inside without her. Several giant globs of the Vicks had made the stench bearable. Not to mention my sinuses were nice and clear.

All throughout the house was garbage. In some areas, garbage was piled to the ceiling. Pathways were carved in the garbage to make it easier to walk through. My glasses were fogging up from the mask, but I could still make out blobs caked onto the carpeting. *Feces - human and otherwise.*

The patient was lying on her side in the kitchen. She was disoriented and moaning, so we couldn't get any information from her. A concerned neighbor was kneeling next to her. The patient's dog was running around, nipping at my ankles. I asked the neighbor to remove the dog. She became indignant. "Why do you care about the dog? Help her! Forget the dog!" *Wow, if she really cared so much for her neighbor, she wouldn't have let her live in her own filth.* I asked her again to remove the dog, which was trying to bite through my boots. She again became angry, so I did the only thing I could... I booted the dog across the room into a pile of garbage bags. "How could you do that?" She screamed. "I would have removed it!" *Tylenol must make a fortune on my headaches at work!*

Without even checking her, we rolled the patient onto the Reeves and carried her out. On the way out, I tripped over a grocery bag. The contents spilled out - dozens of cans of cat food. "That's an awful lot of cat food to be feeding a dog," I commented as I walked out.

"No," the EMT with the Vicks said, "you didn't see all those cats?"

"All those cats?"

Then, as if on cue, dozens of cats began to show themselves throughout the house. They came out from behind garbage bags, looked out windows, climbed on the fence in the back, and lounged on the furniture. I had such tunnel vision I didn't see them. That other component of the stench was cat piss. The EMT knows I'm allergic to cats, you think she would have passed that lil' tidbit of info on to me.

The police met me at the hospital as I was being treated for a violent allergic reaction. They estimated the lady had 100 cats. She couldn't care for herself, but she was able to care for the cats.

A paramedic unit in South Jersey was dispatched for a motor vehicle accident with an unconscious patient on a backwoods road. When they arrived, they saw something that was quite shocking. The man had struck a deer. Judging by the tire tracks, he had slammed on the brakes before hitting the animal. The buck came up over the hood and through the windshield. The deer's antlers became embedded in the man's chest. *Hopefully, the man died instantly.*

When the paramedics tried to assess the man, the deer woke up and started bucking around trying to break free. If the man wasn't dead before, he most certainly was after the deer started trashing about to free itself. *I hope.* The man could not be moved until the police shot the buck and killed it.

The next day, one of the paramedics received a phone call from the medical examiner asking how the patient died. "Isn't it obvious?" The paramedic responded, "The deer came through the windshield and became impaled in his chest."

"It would be obvious," the examiner fired back, "except that he had four slugs in his chest."

The police shot the deer four times, and the bullets passed through the deer and into the man. That would really suck if the deer hadn't killed him.

Dogs bring out the stupid in many people, especially injured dogs. I know that if my dog were injured, I'd probably do something foolish and end up in somebody's book. However, as much as I love dogs, if the injured dog isn't mine, I'm not going near it.

I'm not as heartless as you might believe. One afternoon my partner and I rescued two lost Rotweiller puppies in the park. It was a very hot day, so we gave them water to drink and took them back to the park rangers for safe keeping. We named them Yogi and Boo-Boo.

However, injured dogs are another story. Dying dogs, like dying people, tend to do desperate things. One evening I was returning to my station when I saw a group of people standing in the middle of a highway. They had formed a circle in the road and cars were narrowly getting by without hitting them or each other. I couldn't resist and stopped to check things out.

In the middle of this circle was a dying dog. Hit by a car, its intestines were hanging out on the street. There wasn't much anyone would be able to do for this animal. It was still breathing, but probably not for much longer. The humane thing to do would be to shoot it and put it out of its misery.

"Sir," one teary eyed young man said to, "can't you do anything for him?"

"Yeah, I can call the police and have them come and put the dog down."

"You mean they're going to kill him?" Suddenly I was the most unpopular person there. "You can't just take him to the hospital?" Some people watch too much TV. If I were to bring a dog into the hospital on TV, I'd be seen as a hero and all the women would think I was the cutest and most sensitive man on Earth (*Why can't my life be like TV?*). In real life though, everyone would laugh at me, the department would get fined by the Health Department, the dog would wind up in garbage incinerator, and I would be out of a job.

"No, I can't bring him to the hospital." Growing ever more concerned for the safety of this group, "Why don't we all step out of traffic?"

One valiant young man knelt down beside the dying dog. *My guess is that he was trying to impress the young ladies that were there – heck I probably would have tried the same thing.* He began to stroke the dog's head and let him know that everything would be ok. "What if another car hits him?"

"What if another car hits *you*?"

"Oh, we'll be okay. The drivers can see us just fine." *Famous last words!*

"Dude, you better back away from that dog. Dying dogs can get vicious."

"No, it's okay. Dogs love me."

And as if on cue, the dying pit bull made a lightning fast maneuver and wound up with the young man's arm in his mouth. The dog's death grip lasted until police could come and shoot the dog.

MASS HYSTERIA

Mass hysteria is always good for a laugh. Emergency services usually get very reliable information from the government about how to deal with terrorist attacks or new diseases. *Or at least I can trick myself into believing it's reliable info.* But the general public doesn't always have that info and falls victim to mass hysteria.

In the late 1990's, New York, New Jersey, and Connecticut were introduced to the West Nile Virus. After a handful of elderly people and very young children died from West Nile, everyone began to fear mosquitoes. The symptoms are almost exactly like a cold in the beginning, so throngs of hypochondriacs believed they had encephalitis.

I was called one day for a sick person. When I arrived, a frantic mother nearly ran in front of the ambulance trying to get my attention. She could barely get any words out because she was crying so hard. Finally she screamed "My son has the West Nile Virus!"

I followed her upstairs, curious to see the commotion that would be waiting for us in the apartment. The patient was lying in bed, and very surprised to see us. "Why did she call you?" the twenty-year old man said.

"You have the West Nile Virus, she said."

"What? I just have a cold."

"No!" She began screaming at me. She stormed past me and ran into the kitchen. I feared she would grab a knife and try to kill me. *That would be my luck, wouldn't it?* Instead, she came back with a newspaper and thrust it into my face. "Here! See, it's the West Nile!"

I read the article and saw that it was a list of symptoms. "Ma'am, this sounds just like a cold to me."

"If my son dies, I will sue your asses!"

Being that the son was over eighteen, I decided to let him make the decision to go or not go. He said he would just take Advil and drink juice till he felt better. He signed the refusal form and his mother followed us to the ambulance, yelling and cursing all the while.

A few days later, I was watching an episode of *The Simpsons*, when a preview of the nightly news caught my attention. The first reported West Nile death in New Jersey was reported in Jersey City. I must confess, I was watching with a pit in my stomach, almost convinced that it would turn out to be my patient.

A water main break caused several headaches for my department. Traffic was a mess, fresh water was nowhere to be found, and hysteria was in full force.

I was dispatched for a sick call and found my patient pacing back and forth anxiously in his apartment. "What took you guys so long?"

Ignoring the question, I asked him, "What's wrong?"

"Well, the water main broke and we're supposed to boil the water for ten minutes before we use it." I raised an eyebrow knowing what would come next. "I didn't boil it for ten minutes." *There it was!*

"And are you feeling sick?"

"No, I just didn't boil it all the way."

"You're not nauseous, or dizzy, or having diarrhea?"

"No. But I'm supposed to boil it for ten minutes."

"Well what do you want the hospital to do about it?"

"What will they do?"

"Nothing unless you're sick."

"You mean there's nothing they can do?"

See what I mean? Mass hysteria is fun!

Mass hysteria was in full effect after the attacks on the World Trade Center. In a way it was good. People began taking note of suspicious packages that they would have overlooked before. The bad part was that *everything* was a suspicious package now.

Someone called in a suspicious package at the Jersey City City Hall. City halls present viable terrorist targets, so no one was taking chances. Fire and police blocked off and evacuated the area. The bomb squad came in and set up a robot to check out the package. The package in question was a wheelchair left on the sidewalk near the building with several large packages and bags on it.

As the bomb technician began approaching the package, somehow a homeless man stumbled into the area and walked towards the suspected bomb. SWAT officers tackled the man and dragged him away. The whole time he was screaming, "I need my stuff!"

The technician approached the package and found out that it was nothing more than the homeless man's dirty laundry.

Slightly off the topic...

The same homeless man was my patient several months

later. He was riding the escalator to a PATH station when for some reason he threw his wheelchair down the remaining escalator. He rode the escalator down the rest of the way, then lay down at the bottom and pretended to be hurt. It might have worked had he not been too drunk to realize that the subway station was packed with rush hour commuters who witnessed the whole thing.

I was overflowing with pride following the attacks when everyone placed flags outside their houses or on their cars in support of the firefighters and police officers killed in the attacks. I wanted one for my car too. Of course, I couldn't get a flag without problems. Because I was working so much following the attacks, all the stores I went to on my first day off were sold out. Finally a coworker found a street dealer (*flag dealer* that is) selling flags for $15. I gave my friend the money and he came back with a flag that was one sided. *What the hell kind of flag is* one *sided?*

Finally I managed to find a real flag and proudly taped it to my car antenna. *You knew it couldn't last that long.* Driving home from work one morning, a gust of wind snapped my car antenna in two and the flag flew away in the breeze.

Nearly every ambulance crew adorned their trucks with American flags. A friend went through his own hell trying to find a flag to put on his truck. Finally he found one and displayed it with pride. He went so far as to write on it:

You failed! These colors don't run!

However, much to his disappointment, when it rained for the first time, all the colors in the flag did – red, white, and blue quickly turning into red, pink, and sort of a purplish.

In the wake of the attacks, there were reports of Americans assaulting Arab Americans and robbing their stores. What you didn't hear were the Arab Americans assaulting the Americans. *Hopefully this was an isolated incident.*

Some friends parked their ambulance next to a Dunkin' Donuts and got their ceremonial first cup of coffee of the evening. It was a beautiful night out and they were standing next to the truck checking out the women walking by. The EMTs never realized they were parked across the street from a mosque.

Much to their surprise an angry man came running out of the small mosque. He ran past them and started punching the ambulance and trying to rip off the American flag that was hanging from the mirror. The surprised crew just stood by, watching in disbelief as this man assaulted their truck. Finally, amazement wore off and they called for a supervisor and police. The supervisor was giving the option of sending the man to jail or taking him to the hospital. The supervisor chose to have him admitted to the hospital for a three-day psychiatric evaluation rather than have him released on bail later that night.

I fell victim to mass hysteria myself. This was one of the few times that I have come close to panicking on the ambulance.

We were all mandated to take training in Weapons of Mass Destruction following the 9-11 attacks and the Anthrax attacks. These classes were intended to raise our awareness of what types of weapons could be used by terrorists and how to deal with those attacks. One thing that struck me was how easy it can be to create powerful weapons.

The next shift, after taking these classes, I was dispatched for an assault in an apartment building. When I opened the front door, my partner and I, and the police officers with us began choking and crying. Something in the air was making it almost impossible to breathe. Suddenly my mind filled with images of all the wonderful and nasty things I learned about in class. I was convinced that this was the end.

Luckily for me (and my legions of fans), it was nothing more harmful than OC spray. The patient we were called for had gotten into an argument with his cab driver over the fare. The driver ran him over when the patient got out, then chased the wounded man inside and unloaded OC spray on him. There was so much spray that we had to evacuate the entire building.

Shortly after the 9-11 attacks, someone began launching anthrax attacks, which meant fun on a much larger scale. Never before had we been subjected to such a threat. The cyanide in the aspirin scare of the 1980's had produced a nationwide panic. However, it couldn't hold a candle to the fear and vulnerability we felt with the anthrax attacks. If you didn't buy aspirin, you were okay. However, someone was mailing anthrax.

I sound old saying this, but I remember a time when you would open up a letter and a little white powder would fall out and you'd never think twice about it. Now, people are ever so vigilante about what comes out of their mail.

Some people were logical about it. The chances of a terrorist having enough anthrax to waste by mailing it to *your* house and only infecting one or two people is very slim. Some people, especially in the Mercer County, NJ area, had reason to be concerned because all the letters appeared to have been mailed from the Hamilton Post Office. But some folks let fear and stupidity get the best of them.

Doing my paramedic ride time in Philadelphia, we were dispatched to a furniture store for an anthrax scare. When we arrived, we found out that one of the customers believed she had an anthrax-laced letter. I know what you are thinking, because I was thinking the same thing myself. *What is a customer doing with an anthrax-laced letter in a furniture store?*

Well, this genius checked her mail before she left the house – in New Jersey – and drove across the river to do her shopping. *Don't ask me why she decided to open her mail in a furniture store because I don't know!* She found the first police officer and tried to hand it to him. He did what every police officer in his position would do: he dropped the letter and ran to where he felt was a safe location. I would have done the same thing.

To make a long story short, the powder did not turn out to be Anthrax and the police yelled at her for a very long time.

If you think that was dumb, brace yourself for this!

Later on that same week, we pulled our ambulance into a hospital in Philadelphia. Much to our surprise, there were several fire trucks parked outside of the ER. A lady said she walked outside of her house and found a "white, powdery substance" all over her car.

Now, friends and neighbors, what would you have done in this situation? Being the Monday morning quarterback that I am, I can sit here and say no terrorist would have dumped *that* much anthrax on the car of some unknown person. I would have washed the car and gone about my day.

I'm not saying she didn't have a right to be concerned. Please don't misunderstand me on that. However, again, what would you do? Most logical people who found a potentially hazardous material on their car would turn the other way and find a phone to call the fire department.

She, on the other hand, jumped into the car – *into the hazardous material* – and drove to the hospital. She pulled right into the ER, next to two fire department ambulances, and ran inside. Had this been anthrax, she had just potentially contaminated the two ambulances, the ER, and everyone she passed on her mad dash to the hospital.

When the police investigated the parking space outside of her house, they found nothing to suggest that a powder had been dumped on the car. When the fire department investigated her car, they found no powder. Apparently she had made it all up. In doing so, she took three ambulances, four fire trucks, and several police officers out of service as well as closed down a busy ER for a couple of hours just because she wanted attention.

A friend was dispatched to stand by at an "amtrax" (as it came to be called by many of the callers). The man said he had been opening his mail when he saw a white powder on his envelopes. What tipped off the fire department, and what would have tipped me off as the man opening the mail, was the grease on one of the envelopes. Pizza grease. He was eating his pizza and set it down on the envelopes, and opened the mail when he was done. The powder was nothing more harmful than Parmesan cheese.

Another ambulance was dispatched to a house for an anthrax scare. When the ambulance arrived, the lady who called came running out to meet them with a ZipLock bag in her hands. Inside was an envelope.

"Ma'am, what's the problem?" An EMT asked.

"Well, I just got my student loan papers in the mail."

"Okay, and what's the problem?"

"Well, they come from Trenton."

"Okay?"

"And the anthrax comes from Trenton."

"So?"

"I'm afraid it has anthrax."

"Is there any powder in it?"

"I don't know. I didn't open it yet."

"Then how do you know it has Anthrax?"

"Because it comes from Trenton!"

Hell, I come from Trenton, does that mean…?

Dispatched for a sick person one evening, I found my patient sitting on the couch in the living room of his house. From the zombie-like look on his face, I could tell right away what his problem was. My suspicions were backed up by the broken furniture and TV set.

"You need to take him to hospital. He's not feeling well," his mother said as she got on her clothes to go out to the club that evening.

"He's not feeling well?"

"Yeah, he's acting all crazy. He be breaking furniture and yelling and stuff. I think he gots amthrax."

Completely amazed, I asked her, "Why would you think he has amtrax?"

"Cause, look at the way he's been carrying on. Plus he eats at the fried chicken place down the street and they be putting amtrax in the food down there."

So all those memos from the Department of Defense and the Centers for Disease Control were lying to me. Anthrax doesn't have symptoms similar to the flu – it looks more like PCP abuse.

DUNCAN AVENUE

We're responding for one of my least favorite calls – vaginal bleeding. *Why? Because the patients always seem to be patients you never want to see naked.* But seriously, these calls have the tendency to get messy.

I was never much of a germ-phobic person until I started this job. Mainly, it stemmed from using the public restrooms in the hospitals, and from riding in the elevators in the housing project high-rises.

I give a quick glance around the elevator floor. A broken bottle floats in a puddle of stale urine, surrounded by tiny leaves of marijuana from a smooshed out joint. I pull my shirt over my nose and try to breathe in my cologne through my shirt. It doesn't work quite as well as I hope. I still catch whiffs of the pungent aroma emanating from the little treats on the floor.

The doors open and the hallway is dark and dismal. Graffiti adorns the walls. Much of it would be incomprehensible for an outsider, but I've been around long enough to be able to pick out the ominous artwork of the local gang. My partner and I split up and walk down opposite ends of the hall trying to find the right apartment. The numbers painted on the doors are faded, if there at all. My partner calls and tells me he's got it.

I join up with him and he knocks on the door.

"Who is it?" A voice calls from the other side. I double-check my watch. *It's two in the morning. Who do you think it is?*

"EMS, ma'am."

"Who?"

"Did you call for an ambulance?"

"Yes," she says, still a little unsure of what she should do.

"Then can you open the door for us?" I ask.

We squeeze our way into the apartment, the door barely able to open due to the misplaced couch. I try to give it a shove to get it out of the way, but it doesn't budge. My partner is just able to fit through with the jump bag.

The lady we are following flops down on another couch and says nothing. I look around the room and see no one else. "Um, who are we here for?"

She sighs and flops about on the couch. "Me."

Well, why didn't you just walk out into the hallway with us?

"What's the problem?"

"I'm bleeding."

"Bleeding from where?"

"From down there."

"I see. How long have you been bleeding for?"

"Oh! All day."

I know I'll regret this, but "How long is 'all day?'"

My partner is checking her blood pressure. She thinks about the question, then says, "Since lunchtime."

Lunchtime? That was over twelve hours ago. What made it an emergency now?

"Are you pregnant?"

She snaps her head up and suddenly becomes defensive. "No!"

"Oh, easy. I didn't mean anything by it. I just have to ask." I make a few notes on my clipboard, then ask her, "How is your flow (meaning how is the blood flow)?"

She sits up and looks at me proudly. "Honey, my flo' is so clean you could eat off of it."

And with that, I think it's time we whisk her to the hospital so we can quickly get to making fun of that statement.

MORE SEX INJURIES AND BELOW THE BELT CALAMITIES

It never fails to amaze me what some people do for fun. This chapter might offend some, but I'd let my readers down if I didn't report what I've seen. I'm sorry, but I just gotta tell these!

One of my paramedic instructors was working in Georgia when she was dispatched to a party with chest pain. When she rang the doorbell, a seventy-year old lady answered the door wearing a leather dominatrix outfit. *We can see where this is going already, can't we?*

She explained that her husband was experiencing chest pain upstairs. She led the way up the stairs, exposing the paramedic crew to a view of her butt in a thong.

The patient was lying on the bed complaining of severe crushing chest pain. This they could only make out from his clutching his chest. The patient, an eighty-year old man, was also wearing a full leather outfit, including the mask with a zipper across the mouth.

After cutting away the man's leather clothing, they found out that he had just started taking Viagara and the heat of the outfit, plus a combination of the Viagara and other medications, and the stressful activity on his already once injured heart led him to have another massive heart attack.

I know you're probably looking for some sort of witty comment from me but I won't. I figure that if you live to be that old and you can still get freaky, then I say, "More power to ya!" I would love to be that man when I'm older, *minus the leather mask, of course.*

Actually, I want to be *this* man when I'm older.

A paramedic unit was dispatched for an unconscious patient in a car. When they arrived, they determined that the man who called had been driving around with a dead body in his car for approximately eight hours without knowing the patient was dead.

The man was seventy-five and his 'girlfriend' was sixty-eight. The paramedic unit didn't stick around to find out why the man had been driving around for eight hours with a dead body. However, they were dispatched to return to the scene twenty minutes later for a party with high blood pressure.

When they returned, the man was now the patient. It appears that his wife, who lived around the corner, saw his car surrounded by police officers and came out to check on him. The paramedics found the man on the stretcher in the ambulance, with his wife on the bench next to him, yelling at him, "See, this is what happens when you can't keep it in your pants!"

I want to be like that when I'm in my seventies: have a wife, an active sex life, and driving around for eight hours blissfully unaware that my girlfriend is dead in the seat next to me... Okay, so that didn't come out the way I had hoped. Forget I said anything!

Dispatched to a college dorm for a "domestic entrap-ment," the police wouldn't give us any further information.

When we arrived, we found a young man, naked, handcuffed to the bed in his dorm. He and his girlfriend were playing around with bondage and he said something she didn't like— she left with the key and was nowhere to be found.

In *EMS: The Job of Your Life,* I mentioned how a pre-op transsexual embarrassed me in the ER. I was retelling that story to a couple of friends (No, I won't do it again, you'll just have to pick up my first book.) and one of them blurted out "Oh my god! I know him, or her!

She had the fortune, or misfortune of picking him up for an "injury." She arrived on scene to find the patient doubled over in pain, a towel covering his privates. She convinced him to put down the towel and let her see his injury.

All of the skin around his penis and testicles had been avulsed. "It looked like a photo out of an anatomy book," she told me. He had gotten tired of waiting for the surgery to change his sex and took it upon himself to do it. He took a razor and tried to cut off his stuff. I guess he didn't realize just how involved a surgery such as that really is.

I was dispatched for a patient with abdominal pains. When I arrived on scene, the man was calmly sitting in his living room. He said that his testicles were swollen and painful. Trying to be delicate about the situation, we proceeded with the interview. Then my partner came out and asked, "Sir, do you have boxers or briefs on?"

I don't know where he was going with that line of questioning, but I'm glad I didn't think to ask. The day I ask that is the day I turn in my card.

I was dispatched for another gentleman with "abdominal pain." When I entered his apartment, he asked me if my female partner could wait outside. I told him no and we moved ahead with the questions. He said his testicles were swollen and that they were hurting his back because of how heavy they had gotten.

He stood up and it looked like two grapefruits were stuffed in his underwear. "Can you walk to the truck?"

"Yeah, I think so." What followed next will forever haunt me. He stood up, reached into his sweatpants, and hoisted up his testicles. He walked like that to relieve the pressure on his back. However, when we reached the truck, he took his hand out of his pants and *put it around my shoulder* to give himself a boost.

My partner could not have been more pleased with that. I immediately ripped off my shirt and sped to the hospital. We dumped him off, I changed my shirt, and she began calling everyone on our shift. It wasn't long before everyone was harassing me. "Hey, Dev, you're shirt smells like gonads." "Hey Dev, how does it feel to have a homosexual experience?"

There is no cool way to play off having someone's sweaty mansack on your shirt.

I got her boyfriend back for that. A couple of years later, I responded as a paramedic to a shooting. He was my basic life support. The patient had been shot in the right leg. The bullet entered the thigh, missed anything substantial, exited, and entered the left leg where it blew apart the femur. We "trauma-stripped" the man to check his injuries. I saw what close proximity the bullet had come to striking the man's scrotum. I didn't really feel like checking, so I asked, "Sir, does it feel like your jewels got clipped?"

The patient thought about it. "Nah, man. They feel okay."

Before I could say anything, the EMT in question said, "Well, we gotta check anyway." I watched in disbelief as he checked the man's scrotum for wounds. "They're okay," he said when he finished.

"Bro," I looked at him playing on his homophobia, "I didn't tell you to check. I would have taken his word for it. That means you had a homosexual experience! How does it feel?" I wouldn't have been me if I didn't call and tell everyone on the tour.

I always get frustrated when I'm dispatched to a doctor's office for a pregnant female in labor. *Why do they drive to the doctor instead of to the hospital?* Sometimes you should call the ambulance first, like when your water breaks and the baby is pushing its way through. This woman had the right idea, but failed in the execution.

A woman, who was having her fourth baby, started going into contractions at work. She waited a while, hoping to finish her workday before she had to drive herself to the hospital. On the way, her water broke. She didn't bother to stop at security and ask for a wheelchair, she just continued past and up to the Labor and Delivery floor.

Upstairs, an L&D nurse was waiting for the elevator so she could go down and take her lunch. The doors opened and she almost stepped in without looking. She heard a cry, looked up and saw the baby drop out of the lady.

I'm sorry, but if that were me, I'd be standing there with a look of utter disbelief on my face as the doors closed again and the lady went back downstairs. She would be on her own.

A paramedic unit responded for a gastrointestinal bleed. When they arrived on scene, the BLS were taking down information and getting ready to leave. "What's going on?" One medic asked.

"We would have cancelled you, but you've got to hear this story."

Getting frustrated, the medic responded, "No, I probably don't, but go ahead anyway."

The patient had just gotten out of rehab and was trying to find a way to continue using cocaine without his family finding out. The family knew to look for a red nose, needle marks, etc. So, in his infinite wisdom, the patient came up with a new way to use cocaine by packing as much cocaine as he could into the cap of an aerosol can. When he sprayed the can, cocaine would be expelled. He would aim the can into his rectum and release cocaine inside to be absorbed by the mucous membranes. In theory, it's a very good plan, but something...

That something was the cap!

Somehow it popped off and was lodged in his rectum. In a desperate attempt to remove it, he tried to get up in there with a pair of needle nose pliers. He couldn't find the cap, but he managed to tear apart the linings of his rectum, causing heavy bleeding.

One of the most common responses from patients of rectal bleeds is "*I don't know how that happened.*" It's amazing how no one knows how things got lodged in their asses. The second most common response: "*I fell.*"

An ambulance arrived on a rectal bleed call to find the patient limping around outside. The man was complaining that he had a beer bottle impaled in his rectum. "Sir, how did that happen?"

"I don't know."

The neck of the bottle was inside, with the rest of the bottle sticking out. "Sir, you must know how that happened."

"Okay, I fell off my mantle onto it."

Sure, because everyone has fallen off the mantle while cleaning it, only to fall onto a beer bottle and get it lodged in his or her backdoor. That sounds plausible.

Another crew found their patient was a soup ladle still in his rectum. When interrogated, the patient admitted that he was constipated and tried to scoop out some of his impacted feces with the ladle.

What the hell was he thinking?

This falls under the category of someone who was having a *really* bad day.

A paramedic crew responded at the request of a BLS crew for a head injury and possible leg fracture. When they arrived, the EMTs were bringing the patient out on a backboard. They were also laughing, which is always a fun sign.

The patient, an elderly gentleman, was fed up with listening to his leaky pipes night after night. So that morning he got up, still in his underwear, and leaned under the sink to fix the pipes. His wife's cat, playful as it was, snuck up behind him and swiped at his butt. The cat missed his butt and hit the man's scrotum. In pain, the man jumped and knocked himself out on the pipes above his head. The man's wife was relaying this story to the EMTs at the worst possible time – when they were carrying him down the stairs. They began laughing and dropped the man down the stairs. As he slid down the stairs, the man's foot caught on the railing and broke his leg at the femur.

I really try to remain professional at all times – *honestly, I do.* Sometimes, however, it gets so darn hard!

I was called out for an "unconscious, possible DOA." When I arrived, the BLS and police wore giant smirks on their faces. "Do I really want to know?"

"Oh, yes!" One of the EMTs said. "But I can't tell you, this is just something you need to see for yourself."

I followed him upstairs to the man's bedroom. Before I made visual contact with the patient, the EMT stopped me.

"Hold on, you have to get the whole picture. This is how we found him." He ran over and turned on the TV and VCR. I watched as some very nasty and violent porn came on the TV. The sound was deafening.

"You've got to be kidding me."

"Nope, this is exactly how we found the place!" Over the moans, I asked him to turn it off. I looked on the other side of the bed, and there I found the patient lying on his back with his hand still clamped on his penis. "See what I mean," the EMT said with a beaming smile, "Stiff as a board!"

Like I said, I try to be good, but I can't help myself. "Hey," I called to my partner, "I'll be done in a second. I just need to slap the sticky things on this guy."

Then, it just snowballed from there. Everyone was trying to top each other. "Hey, do you think he had a stroke, or did his heart just peter out?" "Is this going by coming?" "Thank God it wasn't kiddie porn!" The dispatchers were even called, "How are you guys *coming* along?" "Have you completed yet?"

I think my partner won when he called into the doctor to make the official pronouncement. He managed to prompt the doctor to ask, "Is he showing signs of rigor?"

"Oh yes, doc," my partner replied, "he's very stiff."

Thank you ladies and gentlemen, we'll be here all week...

PRINCETON AVENUE AND BROWN PLACE

02:37 hours

The street is dark and quiet, except for the flashing red and white lights of the police cruiser a few blocks up. There is a bright flash of red as the officer strikes a road flare. I pull the ambulance up behind his car and look at the small crowd of people who have gathered to watch.

A station wagon is stopped lengthwise across the street, the front end completely smashed. Doing a quick size-up, I can tell the driver came very fast down the narrow one-way street of Brown Place and slammed into a utility pole. He hit it so hard that he bounced back about five feet. The windshield was cracked on the passenger side. I'm worried that the driver had gone through the windshield, until I see the damage is consistent with the airbag deploying. I whistle with relief as I realize how much worse this could have been. A few inches either way and he would have wound up inside someone's house.

The driver is slumped over the steering wheel and not moving. I can feel my adrenaline rise slightly as I start to think he might not be breathing. As I slip on my gloves, I quickly run through some possible ways to get the patient out in a hurry and what the problems might be. Although it only takes a few seconds, I run through several scenarios at once – multitasking is a benefit of several years on the street.

I reach through the open driver's side window and feel his wrist to check a pulse, all the while I'm keeping an eye for any sign of movement. I don't find one the first time I check, but remaining calm, I feel around to see if I missed it. I find the right spot just as the driver's head snaps back and his eyes fly open. It catches me by surprise and I stumble back into my partner.

The driver lets out a large belch and the cause of the accident becomes abundantly clear. The smell of tequila and beer makes my head spin. The driver kicks open the door and stumbles out, yelling profanities at me as he does so. An empty Corona bottle falls out of the car as he steps out. I notice a half empty one in the cup holder on the driver's door. He grabs my shoulders and starts to say something in Spanish to me. I look at my partner and give him an inquisitive look.

"Bro, I'm stumped." He says to me. "I have no idea what he said."

I push him away, but still he tries to grab my shoulders to talk to me. Fed up, I give him a more than gentle shove and he stumbles back against his car.

"Are you hurt?" A frustrated police officer asks.

The man starts to laugh and mumble in Spanish. He starts dancing a meringue dance by his car.

"I guess that proves he's not hurt," I say in amazement, wondering when this call took such a turn.

The man stops dancing and bends over into his car. He fumbles around for something and that worries the cops.

Both officers draw their guns and start yelling at him to put his hands up. The man laughs and staggers around to face the officers. He tips the Corona bottle he just fished out to the officers and quickly downs the rest of the beer.

"That's it!" One officer holsters his gun and pulls out his handcuffs. "Are you taking him to the hospital?"

"Don't look at me," I say, "I don't give a shit about him." It's hard to feel compassion when all the trouble this guy has caused and *could have* caused.

"Good enough for me. You're under arrest!" He slaps the handcuffs on the man's hands and leads him to the car.

And just like that we are back in service, cancelled by the police. I wish all my calls were this easy.

MOTOR VEHICLE ACCIDENTS

I was dispatched for an "MVA with entrapment" when I was still a junior firefighter and thought it'd be cool because there weren't too many people on the truck and maybe I would get to do something. (Juniors really aren't allowed to do much.)

We arrived (There was already one fire engine on scene.) along with two ambulances, a paramedic unit, and the township's rescue squad. So my hopes of being able to do something useful went down the tubes. Still, being the eager little whacker that I am, I tried to interject myself into the operation wherever I could. I ran back and forth getting blocks of wood to stabilize the vehicle. At first, however, I grabbed the wrong size ones, so the stabilization was off. Once that was corrected, I ran back and forth getting equipment from the ambulance. However, every piece of equipment I got, someone else had already gotten it.

Finally, someone took pity on me and handed me a fire extinguisher. He said, "Stand here and hold this. If it starts to flare up, yell for everyone to move, then pull the pin and spray it down." I figured that would be simple enough. I didn't realize at first just how useless I would be until I saw the hoseline that was stretched off the truck. So I stood there like a complete idiot while they cut the victims out of the car.

When the patients were out and on their way to the hospital, we began the clean-up. I noticed the fire extinguisher had come off of a truck that had left the scene already, so the chief told me to hold onto it until we got back to the station. After cleaning up, I got back on the truck. I lifted the extinguisher up to move it forward, then suddenly learned the hard way that someone had already pulled the pin. With a loud bang, dry chemical powder from the extinguisher shot out and covered the entire cab of the fire truck with a white coating. I opened the door and stepped out, a cloud of white powder kicking up around me. When the cloud dissipated, I could see police officers with their guns drawn, scanning the area to see where the bang had come from. When they realized it was just the idiot covered in white, they put the guns back and began clapping.

For the next several months, I had to endure a ton of harassment. "Hey Dev," they would usually say, "don't feel too bad. Many guys your age suffer from premature or accidental discharge."

My department used to have a policy that if you were driving when you got into an accident, you would have to take a blood test and urine test to check for drugs and alcohol. On top of that, you weren't allowed back to work for the three to four business days it took to get the results back. Notice the phrase "used to." Whenever someone couldn't get approved for a day off, they would just crash the ambulance and go home for a couple of days. It wouldn't be something major; usually we would hit a parked car or clip someone's mirror off. Not a whole lot of damage, no points on our license, and we would get the days off.

Management got smart and changed the policy. Currently, if you get into an accident, you take the drug tests, but you go right back to work and your partner has to drive. The first day they implemented that policy, an ambulance was struck by a car that had run a red light. The EMT driver took the tests, and his partner took over driving. She backed out of the parking space so that could get back in service and backed into a parked car.

Before things changed, I was denied a day off for my birthday. I was trying to think of an excuse not to come in. I was debating whether or not to call out sick, or get sick while I was at work. "Why don't you just hit a parked car," My partner suggested. Right after that, we were dispatched to a motor vehicle accident with entrapment.

I wavered on the idea, but I wanted to make the next job. Not even trying to go fast, I went to make a left turn when I felt something bump into the ambulance and the ambulance bucked. I checked the side mirror to see a small car spinning off across the highway. I pulled over and jumped out. The entire front end of the car had been ripped off. The driver was sitting behind the wheel with a death grip on it, her mouth was moving but no sound was coming out.

I was afraid that I had really hurt this girl. "I didn't even see you there. What happened?"

She managed to compose herself and say, "I pulled out of your way, but then someone in front of me slammed on his breaks and I swerved to avoid him and hit you."

Fabulous! She wasn't hurt, my ambulance surprisingly only had a small dent on it, and now I was all set to get my ticket home for three days.

"I don't know Devin," my tour chief said much to my chagrin. "There's really no damage to your ambulance, so I don't see why you have to go through the trouble of taking the blood test and losing those days."

"No, no chief. Honestly, I don't mind," I protested. "Besides, it wouldn't be fair to everyone else who has to take the test."

"Yeah, but..."

"Chief, no buts! My birthday is tomorrow."

She looked at me and shook her head. "I didn't just hear that. Go get your tests and go home."

Even when I'm not the one in control, things still go awry. It must be me. One snowy evening, I was dispatched to the other side of the county for a life-threatening emergency. I was pissed off because I knew there were closer units available who were just playing games because they didn't want to get more work. Since it was snowing, and since I was pissed off, I told my driver not to kill both of us getting there. Actually, my exact words were "The hell with this! Do the speed limit!" *Why should we put our lives on the line when another ambulance is much closer?*

We were cruising along, cautiously making our way after several cars didn't see us and nearly hit us. After a fifteen-minute trip (and three ambulances dispatched for less life threatening emergencies) we were almost on scene. We approached a red light, slowed down, hit a patch of black ice and slipped right through the light. It wouldn't be my luck unless there was a speeding motorist going through the green light.

My first thought was "Oh my god, we made it through without hitting him." Then *BAM!* The truck spun around and I wound up wedged between the two seats. *Normally I do wear my seatbelt. Of course, the one time I don't...*

I managed to disentangle myself and step out, my shoulder in major pain. The ambulance looked totaled. The front end was banged up and the bumper was hanging on by a thread. The driver of the other car came running up to me and started yelling. "Next time use sirens when you go through an intersection!"

"Hey pal, we slid on some ice. Maybe if you weren't speeding!"

"I wasn't speeding!"

I pointed his attention toward the mangled ambulance. "Sir," I said surprisingly calm, "these ambulances can withstand a twenty-five mile an hour hit. I know that, but more importantly, the cops do, too. So why don't we calm down before I feel the need to press the issue."

There was no need for me to say anything. As soon as the police saw the hit they started grilling him over how fast he was going.

The lady who called 911 had been sick for two weeks with nothing more than the flu. Had been I driving like a maniac, I probably would have made it there with no problem. I can't win!

Dispatched for a "pedestrian struck" call, upon arrival, I nonchalantly made my way to the back of the truck to get equipment. People began yelling at me that I had to do something – which really annoys me. There's no need for me to hurry and risk falling and injuring myself.

As I approached the scene, I started to see that this was indeed a little worse than we were initially told. A bicyclist lay supine in the middle of the street and wasn't moving. All around him was a puddle, which I quickly recognized as blood. One person was holding his head steady, and another was holding a cloth over the man's face and neck.

"Where's he bleeding from?" Everyone shook their heads. No one was sure. My partner and I set about trying to secure the man's airway. He was definitely unconscious. He still had a pulse and was breathing, so we want to pay a little extra time and attention to protecting his airway and neck. I was holding his head steady when someone came and started pushing on my shoulders to get my attention – and at the same time causing me to rock this guy's head all over the place.

"What the fuck do you want?" I finally screamed.

"This man's a doctor!" He began pointing to the man who was holding a rag on the patient's neck.

"You are?" I asked.

"I am?" He said bewilderedly. "I mean, I am. But I'm a pediatrician."

"Perfect." I said, "Keep doing what you're doing."

The same guy who was pushing on my back started trying to get my attention again. "Where are your IVs?"

"We don't have IVs. We're the basic life support. The advanced is on the way."

"Okay, well give me a suture kit. I'm a surgeon."

"We don't have suture kits. Please stand back."

"Well, I've got more experience than you. Let me do something."

Completely frustrated, my partner ripped off the cloth. Blood started pumping straight up in the air. "What are you going to do for *that*?" The bicyclist had been cut off by a car, hit the car, put his head through the window, and then come out again. He had severed his carotid artery and both jugulars on the right side of his neck. He had also avulsed the skin around his trachea, so you could watch it move as he took in breaths.

We managed to package him up and loaded him into the ambulance; where I ran into more obnoxious, self-indulged people. The paramedics muscled us out of the way. "What's his pulse?"

"I didn't count it yet. I just checked to make sure he had one then loaded him up to go."

"Well, how do you know he has one?"

Finally at my wits' end, I waited until the medic was

leaning over the right spot. Then I yanked off the bandage and blood spurted all over his nice white uniform. "Um, he still has a pulse because he's still bleeding," I remarked innocently.

For all the trouble on the call, this was one of the more surprising survival stories of my career (so far). I honestly didn't think he had a chance. His eyes were rolled into the back of his head, and his arms and legs were posturing like his brain had been deprived of too much oxygen. Yet, a few days later, he walked into the police station and got his bike back.

Doctors on the scene can go either way. Some may be helpful, but for the most part, doctors don't have the experience in a setting where everything is out of control. The exceptions to this rule are emergency room doctors.

An ambulance was dispatched for a bad accident on a major New Jersey highway. When they arrived, the crew found that the truck was wrapped around a bridge abutment. The driver had apparently fallen asleep at the wheel and veered off into the concrete pillar. He was driving a truck full of produce. Vegetables and fruit were scattered across the highway.

The driver was in bad shape. He was trapped half in and half out of the truck, unconscious, with one leg amputated below the knee. A motorist had stopped to render aid before the ambulance got there. He identified himself as an ER doctor at a major Philadelphia hospital. He recognized the most serious injury he could help was the arterial bleed from the man's head. The doctor knew he had to apply pressure to the wound, but he found himself with no gloves or bandages. Thinking quickly, he grabbed a piece of lettuce and held that against the man's head until the ambulance arrived. That little bit of produce saved the man's life.

One night when I was working, a couple of guys from the department stopped by on their way out to a club. We were chatting for a little while and they took off. I didn't think much of it until an hour or two later.

We were dispatched for a motor vehicle accident and arrived to find the police had a suspect at gunpoint. Two cars were involved, and both were trashed. Apparently a stolen car had led police on a high-speed chase and ended by crashing into an innocent motorist.

We found the motorist in her car on her cell phone. I tried asking her questions, but she kept dialing numbers and muttering "Why ain't he answering his cell phone?"

I was on the brink of snapping when my partner whispered to me, "Do you know whose girlfriend that is?" I shrugged because I had no idea. He explained to me that her boyfriend was among the guys from the department who went out to pick up women at the club.

"Hey," she asked us, "He's working tonight right?"

Your honor, may I refuse to answer that statement based on the grounds that it will cause bloodshed?

Thinking quickly, I thought up the best answer. "I don't know." *Okay, so I suck when the pressure's on.* "Why don't I have the dispatchers page him?"

We transported her to the hospital for minor injuries. Our dispatchers paged everyone in the group to make sure her boyfriend called back. An hour later, I was bringing someone else to the same hospital. As we pulled in, he was walking into the ER dressed in his work uniform. *Gotta admire a man willing to go the extra mile to cover his lie.*

I was asleep in the station one morning when I was awakened by a loud bang. Even before I looked out the window, I could tell this was going to be a bad accident. A driver had fallen asleep behind the wheel and slammed into a parked car. That car bucked up and landed on her hood, but not before it was forced into another car. That car was forced into another. (That's four in all for those keeping score at home.)

What struck me as odd were the car alarms. All four were blaring and not one of the owners came out to see what all the noise was. *What's the point?*

I was dispatched to the parking lot of a shopping mall during peak holiday shopping season for a car accident. An elderly gentleman had lost control of his car and taken out an *entire* row of parked cars. There had to be at least three cars totaled, and four sustained varying other degrees of damage.

The police had determined that the rug had gotten wedged under the brake and thereby keeping him from stopping the car as he came around a corner. That's something that could happen to anyone, I'm not saying the driver's not at fault, but he certainly didn't deserve the abuse he was getting from the other car owners.

One man in particular was really pissed. As well he should be. I would flip if I came out of Christmas shopping to find my car totaled. He was yelling, "Old people shouldn't be allowed behind the wheel! They are a menace to society!"

I was about to say something when a police officer came over. "Sir, you were driving this car?"

"Yes!" The irate young man said.

Faster than the eye could blink, *click* came the hand-cuffs. "Sir, maybe someone with a warrant for DWI shouldn't evaluate the danger of other drivers."

I couldn't help it. I bust out laughing right in that guy's face. *People in glass houses...*

I responded to a rollover and arrived to find a car wrapped around the guardrail of a major highway. Fortunately, all the occupants were out of the vehicle. The police led one man to us. He was clutching his arm and looking blankly around.

"Hey, man. Like I think my arm is broken."

I took a look and saw that it was obviously broken in at least two places. I quickly assessed the rest of him and found that his arm was his only complaint. I was taken aback that he seemed relatively calm through the whole ordeal. We placed him on a backboard as a precaution and loaded him in the ambulance. I was checked him out further when there was a knock at the door. I opened it and a police officer was standing there, grabbing the arm of another handcuffed youth.

"If this drunk driving piece of shit mattered as a human being, where would you take him?" To accentuate his point, the officer slammed the patient against the side of the truck.

"A trauma center probably."

"Good, I'll see you there." He hauled the young man off and threw him into the back of the police car. *So much for cervical spine protection...*

En route the hospital, I checked over the patient. He was starting to worry me that he registered no pain in the grotesquely deformed arm. "Sir, where you drinking tonight?"

"A little."

"Do any drugs?"

"Smoked a little weed." *Now we're getting somewhere!*

"And did that have PCP in it?

He seemed shocked that I would ask that, like I had just uncovered some major mystery. "How did you know?"

"Because you'd be squealing like a stuck pig right now if you weren't."

At the hospital, he was putting on a show for the nurses and doctors, moving his arm, watching it jiggle back and forth below the breaks.

I was dispatched for an MVA with entrapment and arrived to find the BLS standing by their truck looking into a parking lot. "Any patients?" I asked as I lugged my equipment to the lot.

"We don't know," one EMT answered me. "We can't get close to the car."

I saw that a car had run through a fence and stopped inside the lot. There didn't appear to be any substantial damage to the car and both doors were open. Still we had to check it out. The only problem was the big Rotweiller sitting next to the car.

We stood by for several minutes waiting for a police officer to show up. When they did, the officers approached the dog with guns drawn, just in case. As they walked closer, this vicious beast yawned and rolled over, completely indifferent to the intruders – *hell of a guard dog.* As he did, we saw that the dog was on a chain. Still cautious, the officer shone his flashlight on the dog, which yelped and hid under a pile of garbage.

Really makes you feel like a chicken when you're afraid of a dog who's more afraid of you.

One Thanksgiving morning I responded to a pedestrian struck call. I found the man lying on the ground next to his car. Two firefighters were securing him to a backboard while others were putting the extrication equipment away.

The story we initially got from the patient was that he was working on his car when it rolled off the jacks and hit him. However, the story from several independent witnesses, which was later confirmed by a teary eyed patient, was this: he was working on his car with the vehicle up on blocks. The vehicle kicked loose and pinned him against a wall. He managed to push the car off of him to facilitate an escape. Instead of running for it, he wiped his forehead and said "whew." The car rolled forward again, pinning him once more against the wall.

I'm sorry. That just sucks.

As a paramedic I responded for an MVA with entrapment and found a tanker truck parked on the side of the road. A few feet behind it, off the side of the road in a ditch, was an SUV. As I approached the accident scene on foot, the car burst into flames. Luckily, the patient had managed to get himself out of the car and walked to the ambulance.

We found the man sitting in the back of the ambulance, adamantly proclaiming that he was okay. He didn't want to go to the hospital, despite the massive facial injuries he had. The BLS crew was ready to allow him to sign a refusal, but something just didn't feel right about the situation, so I figured I would talk to him a little more and get a better idea of what was going on.

I asked him a few questions, and became very defensive and evasive in his answers. The man kept saying he had no idea what happened, so I decided not to play around anymore. "You need to go to the hospital. I'll get the cops involved if I have to." With that, he suddenly became cooperative. We were very busy that day, so we decided to do everything en route the hospital. The police said they would meet up with us at the hospital later and finish what they needed to.

"Sir, what is your name?"

"My name is Dave." That struck me as a little odd because he was Egyptian, but I accepted it nonetheless.

"What happened?"

"I don't know."

"Did you fall asleep?"

"No."

"Did you have a seizure?"

"No."

"Did you get knocked out after the accident?"

"No."

"Do you have diabetes?"

"No."

"So what happened?"

"I don't know." At this point I was concerned about a head injury, but more to the point, I felt this guy was just being evasive to cover for something.

My partner had the man's wallet and was searching for his identification. He asked, "Sir, what's your name?" I looked over to see my partner looking at a license with a confused look on his face.

"My name is Dave."

"You sure?"

"Yes!"

"Well, that's not what your license says."

There was a stunned look on the man's face. "Oh, that's what my friends call me. My real name is Osama (that's really what he told me)."

Not wanting to pass up the chance for a good comment, I blurted out, "It's a damn good thing your friends call you Dave." We all had a chuckle, the man even laughed uncomfortably. I proceeded to continue the assessment. "Where do you live?"

"I live in Bayonne."

"Where in Bayonne?"

"I don't know."

"What do you mean you don't know?"

"I just moved in."

"When did you move in?"

"About two weeks ago."

"You've been living in a house for two weeks and you don't know where you live?"

"Why do you keep asking me these questions?"

"Sir, just relax. We have to establish a level of consciousness. Where did you live before?"

"Jersey City."

"Where in Jersey City?"

"(A number) Center Street."

"Dave, the numbers don't go that high on Center Street."

Becoming very defensive, "I meant Central Avenue."

"So you lived at (number) Central Avenue? You sure?"

"Yes!"

"So you mean to tell me you lived at a Dunkin' Donuts?"

He looked at me with the same look of shock as my partner and the BLS crew. "Why do you keep asking me these questions?"

My tapped me on the shoulder. "More importantly, why do you know the address of Dunkin' Donuts?" My partner had more cards in his hands. "I have a question, Dave."

"*What?*"

"Whose car is this?"

"*It's my car!*"

"Don't yell at me Dave, or Osama, or whatever your name is because that's not what the registration says."

Once again, that look of panic and confusion passed across his face. "Ah, um, it's my uncle's car. I'm just borrowing it for today."

I had had enough with the King of Evasiveness for one day. I just started a couple of IVs as a precaution and before I knew it, we were at the hospital. We transferred him to a bed, and on the way out, I ran into one of the cops from the scene. I decided to tell him about the suspicious behavior in the truck. "You guys might want to think about calling the FBI on this guy."

"Oh, why?" The officer said with annoyance as if I were telling him how to do his job. I explained to him that this guy was acting like he was hiding something, and in the post 9-11 world, you can't be too careful with suspicious people. "Well, I'll look in it," he said with an attitude and walked away.

As we got ready to leave, my partner said to me, "Wouldn't it be a pisser if that guy crashed into that truck purposely?"

After we got back to the station, we sat around watching TV. As I usually do, I put on CNN at lunch to catch up on the current events. The lead story was that the FBI had just issued a warning that terrorists might be trying to use tanker trucks as car bombs and that people should be on the alert for possible theft attempts. "No fucking way!" My partner exclaimed as he jumped from his seat.

We hoped in the truck and sped to the hospital. There we found the same police officer. "Did you call the Feds?" I asked.

"You bet I did! Considering what you told us, then this guy gave me three different names, four different addresses, and a completely fake New York State driver's license."

I don't know what came of this, but I'd like to believe that I helped in some small way to foil a terrorist attack.

ARLINGTON AVENUE AND MYRTLE AVENUE

06:09 hours

I groan as I look at my watch. We're responding for another shooting with less than half an hour left in the shift. At this point, I just want to go home. We fall in behind a police radio car and speed effortlessly to the scene.

As we approach, I see half a dozen radio cars blocking off the intersection. Several officers wander around the scene with guns drawn. The Emergency Services Unit officers are once again in full tactical gear. A gun was found on the scene, so they want to be prepared for anything.

I stroll up to the police captain and ask what the story is. They had found a gun and some blood drops, but no patient. We are all ready to pack up and leave when someone calls from the third floor of an apartment building on the corner. "He's up here!"

The ESU officers enter first, guns drawn. We follow close behind, making sure to keep an adequate number of bulletproof vests between us and danger.

The patient is sitting on the couch in the living room as we enter. "What happened?" An ESU officer demands.

"Me and some boys were walking down the street, minding our own business, when these guys start shooting at us."

"Right. How many shots did you hear?" I ask.

"About three."

"How many times were you shot?"

"Just once in my leg." He shows me a small entrance wound in the muscle of his calf.

The police are getting annoyed at this point. They, just like us, are minutes away from shift change. "You weren't doing anything? Then whose gun did we find outside?"

The man begins stuttering. "It's not mine," he finally blurts out. *Good comeback.*

I look at my watch and see that we've wasted ten minutes on this scene. "Where were you shot?"

"Up the block."

"And you walked home and upstairs?"

"Yes."

"Fine, the ambulance is downstairs. Let's go."

Compassion for gangbangers gets thrown out the window at shift change. I just thank goodness my day is finally over. It's time to head home, get some shut-eye, then come back up tonight for some more fun and frivolity.

ASSAULTS

One night I responded for an "unconfirmed" shooting one night, which usually means that someone heard gunshots and called the police to say someone was shot. Most of the time, unconfirmed shootings turn out to be nothing. I was so sure that this one would that I responded eating my ice cream from Dairy Queen.

This time, of course ... I approached the man in the middle of a darkened street to find him lying in a pool of blood. He was mumbling and moving around on the ground, so I knew he was still conscious.

We rolled him over and saw his whole upper body and face were covered in blood. His eyes were still open and following us, so he was still alert and aware of what was going on. "Sir, where are you shot?" I asked as I cut away his shirt to try to find a bullet wound.

His mother was on the scene and she pulled me aside. "He's hard of hearing, but if you talk loud enough he can answer you."

He mumbled something to try to answer me. "Sir, I can't help you if you don't tell me where you're shot." He mumbled something again and by now I was getting very frustrated because I couldn't figure out where he was bleeding from. "Dude, where are you shot?"

"My mouth!" As he yelled that, a large chunk of his tongue fell out of his mouth.

"Holy shit!" I yelled as I sprung back. "That's your tongue! That's not supposed to be there!"

At that point, we hauled ass to the hospital. On the way we were trying to suction out the copious amount of blood that was obstructing his airway. Every so often I had to pull another chunk of tongue out of the suction catheter.

This man was one of the luckiest people I have met. The X-rays showed that a large caliber bullet had entered through his lip, blow apart his tongue, passed through his neck, missed all of the vital blood vessels, and lodged just next to his spine.

The reason he was shot? The shooters held him up and demanded all his money. Because they weren't close enough or talking loud enough, the patient didn't hear them. They figured he was playing tough and shot him.

Why shouldn't you pick up hookers? Besides the fact that it's illegal, and there's that ever-present threat of sexually transmitted diseases, this could happen to you.

A man picked up a hooker one evening and began discussing prices. Once they settled, he paid her. With that out of the way, she pulled out a gun and shot him in the leg. While he was screaming and writhing in pain, she opened his door and pushed him out. Then she made off with his car.

As the EMS crew was patching him up, the police were questioning him. *Now people, there's being honest and being stupid.* Maybe it was the pain, maybe it was the shock of having his car stolen, or maybe he just forgot that he had just done something illegal. He let it all spill out, every last detail. So he got shot, got carjacked, got robbed, and got arrested for soliciting prostitution all in the space of an hour.

Sometimes, EMTs have to go beyond their training and do other functions, including being a therapist, social worker, and in this case, a detective. I responded for a possible DOA. When I arrived, the police officers said to me that it was either a "homicide or a suicide."

I found the patient lying on his bed. He was propped up with his head leaning against the wall, almost in a seated position. From across the room, I could tell he was dead. A small trickle of blood had dried under each nostril. "Why would you think this is either a homicide or a suicide?"

"Did you see the dog?" I shook my head and followed the officer into the kitchen where a German Shepherd was lying on the ground in a puddle of blood. There was a gaping hole in the side of the dog.

I walked back into the bedroom and saw a .357 hand-gun on the patient. At first glance, it might seem like it was a clean cut suicide, except that it was *too clean*.

The dog was lying in a puddle of blood that nearly covered the entire kitchen floor. The man only had a trickle of blood coming from his nose. Also, the gun was *neatly* placed on his chest, pointing directly to his feet. His hands were also *neatly* placed by his side. In order for this to have been suicide, he would have had to have shot himself in the head, then showered, cleaned and shampooed his rugs, neatly placed the gun on his chest, then place his hands by his side and settle in to die.

Once I pointed that out to the police they took the son into custody for questioning.

Here's one of the biggest understatements of all time.

I responded to a shooting and found my patient in the back of a police cruiser – why the officer didn't just run him to the hospital is beyond me. The patient was clutching his hands to his stomach and his shirt was soaked with blood. At first glance we thought he was shot in the stomach. As it turned out, he had his hand blown off when he went to block the gun from going off.

We rushed him to the hospital, and the police officer with us asked him several times if anyone else was with him. He said no. As the doctors were working on him, the officer with us got a call from another officer saying he had found another patient from that shooting.

Being the only unit available, we hurried back into the truck. "Hey," I asked the officer at the hospital, "can you get an update?"

"Sure." He called over and asked for an update.

"We have a twenty-year old male shot multiple times. And Charlie... he don't look too good!"

'He don't look too good?' He was shot six times in the chest. I would hate to see what constitutes *bad.*

An EMT, driving an invalid coach truck, stopped at a hospital to make a pick up. Just before leaving the hospital, he realized he had left his clipboard behind. He pulled around again, got out, and went inside to retrieve the lost item. When he returned, he received the shock of a lifetime. His truck, with his patient, was gone.

Immediately, every police and EMS unit went on the hunt for the missing truck and the patient inside. The patient was a deaf, blind, quadriplegic. Somehow, reports were coming in from all over the city saying that the truck had been sighted at various locations. It was quickly narrowed down to a particular area of the city, and all units in the area converged to come to this patient's rescue.

Meanwhile, on the absolute opposite end of the city, a paramedic unit was clearing up from an assignment when they heard over the police scanner that a radio car had spotted the missing truck literally blocks from the paramedic unit's location. The unit decided to join the chase. As they approached the street where the truck was reportedly seen, they overheard another report that the truck had now flipped over. They turned the corner and sure enough, the stolen invalid coach truck was lying on its side.

The police, charged by the chase, and charged by the fact that some monster had stolen an invalid coach truck with a quadriplegic in the back, jumped onto the side of the overturned truck and ripped the driver out of the truck. The police subsequently manhandled the driver as they yanked him off the truck and dragged him to their car.

The paramedics jumped onto the truck to search for the patient. Much to their surprise, there was no patient inside. Now the situation had gotten even more serious. The patient could have been dumped anywhere in the city.

The paramedic called for a description of the patient. The description came in just as the police were roughly placing the driver into the radio car. Oddly enough, the patient's description fit the driver.

Now the truth came out. A deaf, blind, quadriplegic got tired of waiting for the EMT to come back with the clipboard, so he stole the truck and tried to drive home. He had no idea where he was going, and he couldn't see the police behind him trying to pull him over. Then, the police were wrestling with this man who only possessed 50% strength in the muscles of his body.

The silence of an unusually quiet day was broken by the cries for help from an ambulance crew. Every unit that wasn't doing something immediately sprang into action. Flying from all directions, they met up with the crew in distress.

The driver of the truck was sitting in her seat, but the other crew member was gone. "Where are they?" The responding units demanded.

"He tried to rob us!" She screamed. "He went down that alley!"

Everyone got out of their trucks and took off on foot down a nearby alley. Down the end of this dark alley, the EMT was struggling to keep a young man from climbing over a fence. The man broke free and tried to run past the EMTs. One of them pulled a leather sap out of his back pocket and clubbed the guy in the head, rendering him temporarily incapacitated.

The police showed up and hauled the guy off to the lock up so they could fill out the paperwork. Inside the lock up, the man went through further grilling. The police demanded to know where the money was that he stole from the EMT. "I only have five dollars," he pleaded.

It would be a lie to say that the police did not rough up the man some more. "Where's the fucking money?"

"I only have five dollars!"

The police officer, a close friend of many of the EMTs, was at his wits' end. He was about to use his baton to elicit a better response from the suspect when the EMT who was robbed piped up. "No, that's all he took from me."

Suddenly, everything came to a screeching halt. The officer who was about to beat the suspect dropped his baton in disbelief. "What the hell do you mean that was all? He got an attitude adjustment over five dollars?"

What actually happened was that the man asked for a couple of dollars for gas. The EMT gave him $5 with the stipulation that he would get two dollars back. When it seemed like the man was not going to give back the two dollars, the EMT got out to confront him. *Yes, over two dollars.* The man panicked and ran—at which point the assist was called.

Adding the usual police humor to the situation, the arresting officers photocopied a five dollar bill and faxed it to all the area hospitals with a note on it that read: EMT So-and-So's contribution to Charity Care.

DISPATCHER TALES

In my opinion, dispatchers have the hardest job in the EMS system. They have to remain calm and professional at all times. This is especially hard when the caller is dying on the phone, extremely scared, or belligerent towards the dispatcher. Anyone can pass a dispatcher course, but only certain people can be good at it – *Lord knows, I could never do it!* A good dispatcher can make all the difference in an emergency. The hardest part of their job, as I see it, is that there is a permanent record of what transpires. That means you can't laugh.

These are some actual 9-1-1 calls.

Dispatcher: "911, what is your emergency?"
Caller: "I want to make an obscene phone call."
Dispatcher: "*What?*"
Caller: "I want to make an obscene call."
Dispatcher: "That's what I thought you said. You realize you're calling the police department, don't you?"

Caller: "I know, I want to report a crime, but I don't want to give my name. You know, an obscene phone call."

Dispatcher: "Emergency medical, what is the address?"

Caller: "You know who this is, you motherfucker! I called for an ambulance a half an hour ago and they haven't shown up yet."

Dispatcher: (The dispatcher checked the caller ID and checked the computer screen to see how much time had elapsed since they first received the call.) "Sir, it says you called less that three minutes ago."

Caller: "You asshole! I know I called a half hour ago."

Dispatcher: "Sir, your name is (name) and you're calling from (location)?"

Caller: "Yes."

Dispatcher: "Then you called less than four minutes ago."

Caller: "You motherfucker. You send me an ambulance quicker or I'll come up there and kill you!"

Dispatcher: "Are you threatening me?"

Caller: "I am just telling you to do your fucking job!"

Dispatcher: "My job is to take your call and pass it on to the appropriate agency, and I did that. I can't make the ambulance come any faster."

Caller: "Faggot asshole! I'm going to kick your ass. You get the ambulance down here now or I'll kill you!"

The reason this person was calling? His baby had a fever of 100 degrees.

Dispatcher: "What is your emergency?"

Caller: "This is unbelievable."

Dispatcher: "What is?"

Caller: "I never thought I'd see the day, a UFO in north Lawrence."

Dispatcher: "You mean to tell me you've seen UFOs in south Lawrence? I think I should move."

Dispatcher: "Where do you need the ambulance?"

Caller: "Oh, man, this is horrible."

Dispatcher: "Sir, where do you need the ambulance?"

Caller: "Oh, wow. You gotta see this. This is horrible."

Dispatcher: "What is the problem? And where are you calling from?"

Caller: "You, you just gotta see this."

Dispatcher: "*Sir!* What is the problem and where are you calling from?"

Caller: "Oh gees, you gotta see this, man."

Dispatcher: "Sir, I *can't* see it. But I *can* send someone who can."

Dispatcher: "Emergency medical, where do you need the ambulance?"

Caller: "Yeah, this is security at (a shopping center). We have a prisoner in custody and wonder if you could help us out."

Dispatcher: "Well, what is the problem?"

Caller: "He was arrested for shoplifting shoes and he doesn't have any shoes on right now."

Dispatcher: "So, where do we come in?"

Caller: "We were wondering if you could come down with some of those surgical booties."

Dispatcher: "Sir, you called nine-one-one for this?"

Caller: "Well, can't you just have an ambulance stop by and drop off a pair?"

Dispatcher: "Sir, we are not Payless Shoes. We do not do things like that."

Here's where I probably would have lost it and gotten fired for cursing someone out on the phone:

Dispatcher: "Emergency medical, what is the address?"

Caller: "Yes, I'm calling from (location) and I have an emergency."

Dispatcher: "What is the problem?"

Caller: "Well, my daughter is stuck in her car and..."

Dispatcher: "You're daughter's stuck in her car? Do you need the fire department?"

Caller: "Not like that. She needs to get out and there are ambulances and fire trucks blocking her in."

Dispatcher: "Is this an emergency?"

Caller: "Yes, it is. She needs to get out and she called me in tears."

Dispatcher: "Does she need us to send her an ambulance?"

Caller: "No, she doesn't need an ambulance."

Dispatcher: "Then why did you call nine-one-one?"

Caller: "Can't you call the ambulance and have them move their truck?"

Dispatcher: "Ma'am, they have someone in cardiac arrest they are working on. They should be out in a little while."

Caller: "Well, can't someone just come down and move the truck? Do they need all those people in the apartment?"

Dispatcher: "Ma'am, I am not going to have them stop what they are doing just so that your daughter can get out. Unless she needs an ambulance, it's not really an emergency."

Caller: "Well, I just hope the ambulance is okay when they come out."

Dispatcher: "What is the emergency?"

Caller: "You guys owe me a dollar fifty."

Dispatcher: "Sir?"

Caller: "This pay phone took my money and won't let me call."

Dispatcher: "Okay, sir, you called an emergency number. You need to hang up and call the phone company."

Caller: "But the sign here says for emergencies I should call this number."

Dispatcher: "I understand that sir, but this is not an emergency."

Caller: "How do you know? I need to use the phone. It's an emergency to me. You guys owe me a dollar fifty."

Dispatcher: "What is the emergency?"

Caller: "I'm calling from (location). Someone just jumped off of the eighteenth floor."

Dispatcher: (With an air of disbelief) "Really? How do you know he jumped off the *eighteenth* floor?"

Caller: "Cause I'm on the seventeenth and he just dropped past my window."

A group of co-workers were going through the training for dispatcher. They were a tight bunch, so they had a lot of fun together. One day at lunch, they decided to have a few drinks before heading back to class. One of them had a little too much, and that afternoon they were supposed to do simulated phone calls.

Caller: "Hello. My baby's not breathing!"

Dispatcher: "*Really?* Are you sure she's not breathing?"

Caller: "Yes! She's turning blue!"

Dispatcher: "Ah! Wonderful. *Wonderful!*"

Dispatcher: "Emergency medical, what's the address?"

Caller: "I'm calling from (address)."

Dispatcher: "Okay, ma'am what is the problem?"

Caller: "I have vampires living in my attic..."

Dispatcher: "Wait, ma'am, you have *what* in your attic?"

Caller: "Vampires!"

Dispatcher: "Okay, ma'am how long have you had these vampires in your attic?"

Caller: "A very long time."

Dispatcher: "So what made you want to call me about these vampires tonight?"

Caller: "Because they want to come down and fuck me in the ass tonight!"

Dispatcher: "Okay, I can see how that's an emergency. We'll be sending the police on the double."

★ *The name has been changed*

Dispatcher: "Sir, are you calling from (location)."

Caller: "No, I'm calling from (exact same location the dispatcher said)."

Dispatcher: "That's what I just said. What is your name?"

Caller: "Mister Johnson★."

Dispatcher: "Sir, what is your first name?"

Caller: "Mister."

Dispatcher: "No sir, what is your first name."

Caller: "Mister."

Dispatcher: "Okay, let's try this. How do you spell your first name?"

Caller: "M-I-S-T-E-R!"

Dispatcher: "Where is the emergency?"

Caller: (Loud sipping sound) "Ahh, I need an ambulance."

Dispatcher: "Why do you need an ambulance?"

Caller: "I'm not feeling well."

Dispatcher: "What do you mean, you're not feeling well?"

Caller: (Another sipping sound) "I need detox."

Dispatcher: "You need detox? And you're drinking while you're on the phone with me?"

Caller: (mumbles something incomprehensible)...

Dispatcher: "What was that, ma'am?"

Caller: (sipping again, followed by mutter)

Dispatcher: "Ma'am, put the forty down while you talk to me."

Caller: (sipping, followed by crashing and glass breaking) "Oh shit!"

Dispatcher: "Ma'am?" *No response.* "Ma'am, are you

there?" *Still no response.* "Ma'am, what happened?"

Caller: "Ah damn it. That was a fine bottle of Thunderbird! I paid a buck-eighty for that!"

Caller: "I called for an ambulance several minutes ago and I want to know why they haven't come up yet!"

Dispatcher: "Where are you calling from?"

Caller: "I'm calling from (location), apartment 4-D."

Dispatcher: "Ma'am, according to the computer, that ambulance should be off by now."

Caller: "I know they're here, but I want to know why they haven't come up!"

Dispatcher: "What do you mean?"

The caller opened the window, hung the phone out, and over the unmistakable sound of an ambulance PA, one could hear, "Will the caller in apartment 4-D please walk your asthmatic grandmother downstairs?"

SILLY HUMAN TRICKS
AND OTHER
MISCELLANEOUS STORIES

I know I'm allergic to certain things, such as cats and latex, and try to avoid them at all cost. Why is that so hard to understand? I worked a severe allergic reaction one afternoon. The patient was so severe we had to intubate him and he spent several days on a vent. He knew he was allergic to peanuts. Guess what the BLS found in his lap? That's right, a can of mixed nuts!

Driving back to the station one evening, my partner turned to me quickly and said, "Hey Dev, is that smoke?" He pointed down the street, and sure enough, a thick layer of smoke was wafting across the street.

I decided not to call it in until we figured out where it was coming from. We passed in front of an elementary school and found the dumpster was on fire. There was a man in shorts and flip-flips, standing in the dumpster trying to stomp it out.

"Three-Oh-Five to Dispatch," I called in, "notify FD that there is a dumpster fire on the corner of Kennedy and Broadman. We'll be standing by for them."

"Five, why do you need to be there?"

"Because there's an idiot in flip-flops and shorts trying to stomp it out."

"Understood, sir."

As we got out of the truck, the man packed up and ran off, leaving the dumpster to burn. Feeling a wave of civic duty, I grabbed the fire extinguisher off the ambulance and sprayed down the dumpster. I knocked it down and felt pretty damn good about myself.

Here's an important thing to remember about fire extinguishers: check to see what types of fires the extinguisher can put out. I was under the impression that most extinguishers could put out normal fires, or those that burn things like wood or paper. Well, as it turns out, this extinguisher could put out electric fires and fires with flammable liquids, but not an ordinary trash fire. *I know. That makes no sense to me either.*

I sprayed it down, thought it was out, went to go check it out, and the fire flamed up again. This time it was worse than before. You know, you try to do a good thing and it comes back to burn you in the ass. *Literally.*

Here's how pathetic I was in high school:

I was dispatched to my first fire while volunteering with the first aid squad. We were dispatched to stand by. It was in mid September, but still warm and humid, so we could tell it was going to be busy.

The fire was in a book depository on the campus of a large prep school. There were two main entrances into this school, and of course, on this evening we chose the wrong one. After driving aimlessly through the campus for more than ten minutes, we finally saw the flashing lights of many fire trucks. When we made our way over, we became aware that if we had taken the other entrance, we would have been right at the fire. Oh well, that's me: the king of bad directions.

Not a whole lot was happening at first, so I decided to occupy my time by checking out the crowd. I noticed that there were many high school girls watching the fire, which was good for me since I was a high school guy. So I started to feel pretty cool, granted I had no reason to, but I felt that these girls were checking me out nonetheless. *Hey baby, you like guys in uniform?* My friend Ray, another junior, came over and made the same observation. Those girls were checking us out.

With my ego inflated, and my head filled with visions of actually walking up to one of them and striking up a conversation, I didn't hear the fire chief screaming for an ambulance. In fact, I didn't notice I was needed until I looked around and saw the crew run off without me. I took off after them, running madly.

Out of breath, I stopped next to my partners and asked the chief where the patient was. "Ah, Dev" he said nervously, "you're standing on him." I looked down and, sure enough, there was an unconscious firefighter lying on the ground with me standing on his hand. I quickly got off before the firefighter could register pain, and began treatment. He was followed by another firefighter with heat exhaustion, then another, and another, until with had fourteen firefighters in the treatment area.

Starting to become frantic because I had never been faced with more than three patients before this moment, I ran back to the truck to get more supplies.

Seeing firefighters and EMTs running around frantically made the crowd want to watch closer, as if they knew something was wrong. As I ran for the truck, I could feel dozens of eyes on me, studying my every move. *Yes,* I thought, *dozens of babes are checking me out. Can't let them see me screw up.*

Well, as if saying that made it come true, I tripped over a curb. I hadn't fallen flat on my face yet, and I was yelling at myself not to fall. But, just when I thought that I would make it out okay, I tripped over my own feet and fell. I could feel pain shooting through my knees and warm blood trickling down my wrists from the scraps on my palms. Then, to rub salt in my wounds, I could hear people in the crowd laughing at me. It was probably the most embarrassed I had felt in a very long time.

But at least I wasn't alone. My friend told me later that he was told to go back to the truck and get another length of supply hose, and run it to the ladder truck—a simple enough task, and one that would have run in full view of a group of girls. Well, he got a little too excited, grabbed the hose and ran for the ladder truck. The idea was that, by running, the girls might think you were important. Due to the noise of the engine and the pump, he didn't hear that the hose was (1) not the right hose he was told to get, and (2) still attached to the hose reel. He made it fifty feet when he ran out of slack. It snapped back and knocked him on his ass in front of a crowd of laughing girls.

Man, was I sad back then or what? Not much as changed, but at least I can laugh about it. That taught me to pay more attention to the task at hand, and not who was watching.

For a working structure fire in Lawrenceville, I was on one of the last trucks to make it to the scene. All of the occupants were out of the house. Everyone except Fluffy, the family dog.

I was assigned to search the basement with another firefighter to locate the dog. I'm a dog lover, but I find it a little odd to send people into the floor *below* a fire to look for a dog that is probably already dead. If it were my dog, sure, I'd do it in a heartbeat. This wasn't even a cool dog like a Rotweiller or golden retriever. It was a miniature dog, one of those yippy rat dogs. I doubted if I could even find it.

We forced our way into the completely black basement by cutting open the storm door in the back of the house. I didn't have my contacts on that day, so I misjudged how close I was to the opening. I tripped down five concrete steps, somehow ripping up my leg without damaging my brand new turn out gear.

We began crawling around on our hands and knees trying to find this rat. The only light we had was the smoke muffled beam from the flashlight. The smart-ass that I was sent down with decided he was going to have a little fun. He picked up a stuffed teddy bear and tossed it over my shoulder. "Hey, I think that's Fluffy!" he screamed.

I was so excited. I didn't want to be right under the fire looking for a dog. I reached out, felt it, and jumped up to turn around and head out. I didn't realize that I had crawled under a table. I whacked my head hard enough to knock my helmet off. This guy is laughing his ass off at me. I felt pretty damn stupid. It would have been like that scene in *Backdraft* where the guy brings out the mannequin.

How's this for justice? It's probably wrong to laugh at this, but considering what these guys did...

In some of the housing projects, the kids like to "Elevator Surf." They ride on the outside of the elevator cars, and when they get the feeling, they flip the hatch open on the top of the car and urinate on the people inside. I've heard about them pissing on cops, firefighters, and EMTs who where unlucky enough to be riding in the cars.

One afternoon, a young man was dared by his friends to do it. He was riding the roof of the car, flipped the hatch, and began to pee on the wrong lady. She hit the emergency stop bottom so fast that it knocked the kid off the elevator and wedged him between the car and the wall. When the fire department arrived to free him, he had pissed himself again.

Another prodigy of the housing projects thought he had the ultimate drug business going. He would sell heroin from his building, but the police could never find his stash. He taped large amounts of heroin to the underside of the elevators. The elevators in the building stop at every other floor. To get to his stash, he would have a friend stop the odd floor elevator between the 5th and 3rd floors. He would open the door on the 3rd floor, reach up and grab the dope.

His scheme worked for a while, but only because he was very lucky. He didn't realize, or didn't care, that you need to cut the power off to the elevator cars if you want to carry out a plan such as this. He took too long trying to get the heroin out from under the car one day, and someone on the ground floor called for the elevator. The car started down, and before he knew it, the elevator had decapitated him.

Being able to express yourself clearly is an important trait for an EMT. I like to think I'm a good talker – I kissed the Blarney Stone! I have a talent for being able to talk just about anyone into going to the hospital and calming down frantic patients or family members. However, I, like many others, find myself saying the wrong thing to my patients without thinking of it.

Early on in my volunteer career, I had an elderly female who was having chest pain. We assessed her, packaged her up, and brought her out to the ambulance without a problem. Once inside the ambulance, the county paramedics arrived and began their assessment. They were listening to her lungs and asking other questions. One paramedic asked me what her pulse was.

Trying to sound smart, I said, "She's very tachy." *Meaning she's tachycardic, or her heart is beating very rapidly.*

The lady gave me a very indignant look and said, "Excuse me! I may be many things, but I am *not* tacky!"

I was attending to an elderly patient who wasn't feeling well. For the past couple of days she had been experiencing flu-like symptoms. She exhibited no life-threatening signs or symptoms, so I didn't think it was that big a deal.

"Okay ma'am, we'll take you over to the hospital and get you checked out." I gave her a smile and guided her by the arm to the stretcher. As soon as she started to walk, she began to cry. "What's wrong?"

"I wish my daughter were here with me."

I clued into what she was saying and told her everything would be okay. My partner, on the other hand, didn't realize what she was saying. "That's okay ma'am, your daughter called and said she'd meet us at the hospital."

She began wailing uncontrollably. "No! My daughter died three years ago."

A man was running late at work. As such, he got to the PATH station just as the subway train was pulling out. Thinking quickly, he tried to jump onto the moving train.

Predictably, since this is the Silly Human Tricks chapter, he missed. He became tangled in some wires and was dragged about twenty feet or so before the train stopped. Luckily the train had just left and hadn't had the chance to speed up.

When we arrived, the patient was crying hysterically. We checked him out and found that he wasn't in any immediate danger. We packaged him up and started moving to the ambulance. He continued to cry and plead with us. "Don't tell anyone what happened. In my country (Japan) this is very shameful."

My partner looked at him with a serious face, "Don't worry. This is the good old US of A. And this is *still* shameful here."

THINGS I JUST DON'T UNDERSTAND

"Do you have any medical problems?"

"No."

"Do you take any medications?"

"Yes, I'm on Dilantin and Phenobarbital."

"So you have seizures?"

"Yes."

"Then that's a medical problem."

It's frustrating when you're trying to assess a patient and they're never forward about their medical history. It never fails. I ask the patient what medical problems they have and they say none. Yet, when I ask them what medications they take, they give me a list a mile long.

Part of it could be ignorance, but there is no excuse for not knowing about the meds you're taking. Something's not right with you, you go to the doctor. The doctor then gives you a prescription and tells you to take one of these every day for the rest of your natural life. Am I the only person who would think to say, "Oh, no. Doctor what's wrong with me?"

I have no problem with a person not knowing all the medications they are on if they take a lot. But at least know *why* you're on these meds.

Babies with fevers

A common call is the baby with a fever. Apparently no one has heard of a private doctor, but that's beside the point. I see nothing wrong calling an ambulance if your baby has a fever of, say 102 degrees and *your baby is seizing*. I know that I'll be flipping out every time my kids cough when I have them. But if you are going to call the ambulance because you *think* you're baby has a fever, *check* the baby's fever.

"What's the matter?"

"My baby has a fever."

"How high?"

"I don't know."

"Then how do you know it's high?"

"She feels warm."

"She feels warm because it's hotter than an oven in this apartment."

Why would you call 911 because your baby has a fever? There is nothing I can do that would change it, and you're not going to get into the emergency room any faster unless the child has a seizure because of the fever, but that's a whole other ball of wax. I get quite angry when I walk into the house and there are at least 5 people who have drivers' licenses. *Take your own car and save a few hundred bucks!*

And while I am on the topic, is it so hard for you to be ready when I get there? You call 911 because the baby has a fever that won't go away. So the fever's been there for at least a few hours. Once you call, it usually takes us about seven to eight minutes to make it to your house. *What do you do in that time that you couldn't throw some clean clothes on the kid?*

Also, *is it so hard for you to be waiting at the front door when I get there?* I can't begin to tell you how many times the mother comes downstairs to open the door then walks us back up four flights of stairs to get the child who is sitting on the bed waiting to leave. *Bring the kid with you when you let us in and save us all some walking!*

Rubbing Alcohol cures nothing!
I know many people were brought up believing in the old wives' tale that rubbing alcohol will cure most common ailments. Now we have the problem of mothers submerging their children in rubbing alcohol when they have a fever. Now the kid still has the fever and is pickled inside.

If rubbing alcohol cured everything, why would I be carrying hundreds of thousands of dollars worth of equipment in my ambulance? Why would I have to go to school for four months to become an EMT? Wouldn't my truck be stocked with $0.99 bottles of alcohol?

I was trying to assess a man who was having a heart attack. As he was struggling to breathe, his wife kept pushing me aside to rub alcohol on him. "Ma'am, stop doing that," I told her politely.

"Ignorant motherfucker," she responded, "what if he dies?"

Good comeback. Didn't see that one coming. I had a good mind to let her continue so that when I went to defibrillate him he'd light up like a Christmas tree.

While on the subject of rubbing alcohol, I passed a convenience store in a part of town that was populated with a large congregation of our regular drunk patients. There was a sign in front of the store that read **24 oz. Alcohol, $0.99 a bottle**. *How much misunderstanding do you think that caused?*

Unknown Medical Emergencies

I can't understand why I get dispatched for unknown medical emergencies. When you dial 911, can't you give me some idea as to why you called for my services? "*I don't know*" is not an appropriate response to the 911 operator asking what the emergency is.

Obviously something happened that made you feel the urge to call 911, so tell me what it is. I'm not asking to delve into the root cause of the problem, but if you called because you found some guy not moving on the sidewalk, tell the dispatcher that. If you called because there is a woman yelling and screaming that she has a knife and wants to stab someone, tell the 911 operator that so I don't find out the hard way.

Self-Schooled Traumatologists

Just because you watch *ER* or re-runs of *Emergency* does not mean you are qualified to tell me how to do my job. Granted, if a child has some sort of medical problem that requires specialized equipment, like a ventilator, I can guarantee that his parents know more about what is going on than I do. So I use that to my advantage.

However, if someone is hit by a car or shot or having a heart attack, unless you have EMT or better before or after your name, don't stand over my shoulder and tell me what I have to do. I don't have to hurry. I don't have to give him medications, and I don't need to "be doing something." In fact, the only thing I need to do is pay taxes and die, and there are probably ways around the taxes part. Stand back, keep your opinions to yourself, and let me work so I can help this person.

Have some faith that I know what I am talking about. People are so quick to become defensive and hostile when you point out the basic flaws in their medical beliefs. I had a patient complaining of a nosebleed because of her high blood pressure. When I tried to start an IV on her, she told me she was allergic to salt water. When I inquired further she told me her doctor told her to stay on a low salt diet and demanded I not start the IV.

Allow us to eat

Ambulance personnel work hard. Some of us aren't even allowed an hour lunch break. If you see an ambulance crew eating, leave them alone. Unless you are going to thank them for the job that they do, just let them be. It is such a slap in the face when I spend all day racing around town and being submerged up to my elbows in blood and vomit that some people still have the urge to harass me when I try to get something to eat.

"Why are you in here eating when people out there are having heart attacks?"

Because dumb ass, if I'm in here eating that means they haven't called yet. And I'm certainly not one to go door-to-door asking if everyone's okay before I sit down to eat my meal.

"My dog doesn't bite."

Your dog doesn't bite *you*. To him, I look like a doggy treat with a blue uniform on. And as dumb as some people think dogs are, you can't lie to a dog when its master is hurt. You can lie to the family, but the dog knows something's up. And if the master is in pain, and I try to go near him, the dog will assume that I am trying to cause him further harm, and try to defend its master.

Please lock the dog up in the other room when we ask you to. Yes, your dog is cute, but not when he latches onto my leg and tries to make a meal out of me.

The ambulance is not your taxi.

I could be wrong, but I do believe there is no law that says I am obligated to drive you from one hospital to another just because you are unhappy with how fast that emergency room staff is working. *Have patience. If you're in the waiting room, then the staff does not feel you are an emergency. And trust me, the staff at the other hospital will think you even less of an emergency when I tell them where I picked you up.*

The ambulance is not here just *for* you.

The ambulance is there to be used by everyone in that community. So if the ambulance is slow to respond to your call, it may be busy with another patient, or has been redirected to a call in which another patient is in worse shape than you.

Things happen on a daily basis that we don't have control over. We do our best to respond to these situations and to overcome them. I try my hardest to keep my ambulance clean and smelling good.

I once had a patient who was horribly burned in an explosion. We worked on him for a half an hour in the ambulance trying to start IVs so we could give him some morphine and to intubate him so we could control his airway. It took me an hour and a half to clean up my ambulance. I wish I could have had longer to work on it, but I was rushed out of the station for a baby with a fever call that had been holding for twenty minutes.

There is the first part of this problem, *why would you wait almost a half hour for an ambulance when you could drive yourself or call a taxi?* When we arrived, the mother was upset that she had to wait so long. Then when we got her in the back of the truck, she began to complain about the smell of burnt flesh. "Why's it smell so nasty back here?"

"Because lady, the guy before you had a *real* emergency."

People who cannot walk never seem to be on the first floor.

I can't understand why people put relatives with serious medical problems in the most inaccessible areas of their houses. They'll move the relative into a back bedroom, but move everything from the bedroom into the hallway making it next to impossible to fit through. The relative is always getting sick, and the ambulance is always getting called, but the family never thinks to move the garbage out of the hallway.

Plus, why can't you move them to the first floor of the house when you know you'll be calling an ambulance for them constantly? Make it easy on everyone. We don't like carrying people because it's dangerous; we could fall or injure our backs in the process. And lord knows the patient doesn't like to be carried. It's a scary thing to have someone carrying you down a couple of flights of stairs. So have a heart and move them to the first floor, please.

Also, if you are considered on the heavy side and have serious medical problems, like asthma or something else that would require you to be visited by the friendly neighborhood ambulance on a frequent basis, move downstairs.

I had a patient who, at the risk of sounding cruel, was so large that she looked like they built the room around her. She was having an asthma attack in a second floor bedroom that barely fit the bed in it. There was no way we could carry her out because the way the furniture was arranged we couldn't fit a carrying device in. Also, because the room faced another building, we couldn't have the fire department cut through the wall to lower her out that way. The only thing we could do was to give her Albuterol breathing treatments until she cleared up and walk her to where we could put her in some type of carrying device. We gave two treatments and walked her three feet. She had another asthma attack. We sat her down, gave her two more, she cleared up, and we walked her three more feet, where upon she had another asthma attack. By the time we got her to the hospital, she had gotten nine treatments, the standard dose is usually two to three, and her heart rate was about 160 because of the Albuterol. Most of this could have been avoided if she lived on the first floor.

We joke sometimes and say there is a direct correlation between what floor the patient is on and how much they weigh, one hundred pounds per floor. I once backed up another ambulance with a lift assist because they had a large patient. They were on the fourth floor, and sure enough their patient weighted over four hundred pounds. We had to get the fire department to send two fire trucks to assist us. We strapped her to large plank of wood and lowered her down the stairs using twelve people. At one point, she moved. Someone at the top lost his balance and slipped, my partner dislocated his shoulder, the wood slipped and landed right on my foot. Thank god for steel toed boots, but it still hurt like hell. Everyone was concerned about my partner and no one was paying attention to me. I started yelling for help, "Guys! Help! Guys! Fat woman on my foot! Fat woman on my foot!"

Walking back inside.
Probably my biggest pet peeve is when a call happens on the outside, and magically the patient appears on the third floor and now needs to be carried down. *Just stay outside!* You know you're going to the hospital, so why add extra work? It is a pain in the butt to walk upstairs with all our equipment, only to have to walk down with all the equipment and the patient.

More annoying than that, is when a patient calls for the ambulance because they are sick or experiencing something they perceive to be an emergency, then walks downstairs to answer the door, only walk back upstairs and flop down on the couch. If you know you're going to the hospital, and can walk down the stairs, bring your keys with you and save a step.

Why the hostility?

The last time I checked, EMTs helped people. Wouldn't that make us the good guys? So why are people hostile towards us when *they* called for us?

It never fails to amaze me that someone could call 911 for someone they perceive to be an emergency, and then be belligerent towards us when we arrive. I can understand if someone else calls for you and you wanted nothing to do with the ambulance. However, there are people that call for themselves and then get angry at the crew the second they walk through the door. *Where's the love?*

I had a patient call 911, and the moment I got into her apartment, she began yelling, "You ain't shit!" Then she demanded I get her bottle of vodka off the shelf in the other room. I'm sorry, but I missed the bartending classes in EMT and Paramedic school.

The things that make this job stressful and frustrating are also what   make it so interesting. We are called upon to do so much more than we are trained to do. Not many other jobs can say that. On any given call, we may have to be a psychologist, a social worker, a police officer, a babysitter, a taxi driver, a therapist, a teacher, a construction worker, or a host of other jobs and professions.

As long as this job stays interesting, I'll be doing it. And as long as I stay a magnet for strange and unusual events, you'll be reading about it.

Stay safe out there!
Devin Kerins
Liberty State Park,
Jersey City, NJ
June 14, 2004